D1377718

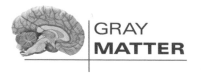
GRAY
MATTER

The Midbrain

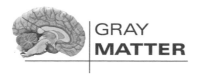

GRAY
MATTER

Brain Disorders
Cells of the Nervous System
The Forebrain
The Hindbrain
Learning and Memory
Meditation and Hypnosis
The Midbrain
The Neurobiology of Addiction
Sleep and Dreaming
The Spinal Cord

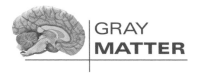

GRAY
MATTER

The Midbrain

Michael Morgan

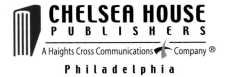

CHELSEA HOUSE
PUBLISHERS
A Haights Cross Communications ✦ Company ®
Philadelphia

CHELSEA HOUSE PUBLISHERS

VP, NEW PRODUCT DEVELOPMENT Sally Cheney
DIRECTOR OF PRODUCTION Kim Shinners
CREATIVE MANAGER Takeshi Takahashi
MANUFACTURING MANAGER Diann Grasse
PRODUCTION EDITOR Noelle Nardone
PHOTO EDITOR Sarah Bloom

STAFF FOR THE MIDBRAIN

PROJECT MANAGEMENT Dovetail Content Solutions
PROJECT MANAGER Pat Mrozek
PHOTO/ART EDITOR Carol Field
SERIES AND COVER DESIGNER Terry Mallon
LAYOUT Maryland Composition Company, Inc.

A Haights Cross Communications ✦ Company ®

www.chelseahouse.com

First Printing

10 9 8 7 6 5 4 3 2 1

Library of Congress Cataloging-in-Publication Data

Morgan, Michael, 1960–
     The midbrain / Michael Morgan.
     p. cm. — (Gray Matter)
Includes bibliographical references and index.
     ISBN 0-7910-8637-2
1. Mesencephalon. I. Title. II. Series.
QP378.M67 2005
612.8´264—dc22   2005011988

All links, web addresses, and Internet search term were checked and verified to be correct at
the time of publication. Because of the dynamic nature of the web, some addresses and links
may have changed since publication and may no longer be valid.

Contents

1. Don't Overlook Me! 1

2. Comparative Neuroanatomy: Is Bigger Better? 13

3. Movement: Two Colorful Nuclei 23

4. The Impressive Inferior Colliculus 35

5. Seeing Without Believing 50

6. Defense: The Real Story of *Survivor* 64

7. Reward: Sex, Drugs, and Rock 'n' Roll 78

8. Fibers: Before the Wireless Revolution 90

Glossary 99

Bibliography 105

Further Reading 106

Web Sites 107

Index 108

1 | Don't Overlook Me!

Do you feel overlooked, underappreciated, or taken for granted? If so, then you can relate to the plight of the midbrain. The cerebral cortex gets most of the attention while the midbrain does its work in relative obscurity. Even the relatively simple spinal cord gets more attention than the midbrain. However, if you take the time to get to know the midbrain, a fascinating and vital part of the nervous system will be revealed. The chapters of this book will explore the secrets of the midbrain from sensory and motor processing (Chapters 3, 4, and 5) to complex behaviors such as defense (Chapter 6) and reward (Chapter 7).

The terms forebrain, midbrain, and hindbrain are descriptive labels for different parts of the brain. These names provide anatomical, not functional, information about the brain. The forebrain is in the front and top, the midbrain is in the middle, and the hindbrain is at the bottom of the brain. Although forebrain, midbrain, and hindbrain are part of a common labeling scheme, it is not the only one. For example, the hindbrain is called the metencephalon, the midbrain is called the mesencephalon, and the forebrain is made up of the diencephalon (**thalamus** and **hypothalamus**) and telencephalon (**cerebral cortex** and **basal ganglia**). Names take on a functional significance when identifying the many anatomical structures located within the brain.

BRAIN ANATOMY

Enter the anatomy laboratory of a medical school and you will find yourself surrounded by well-preserved dead humans covered by blankets. Remove the top of the skull and the brain will appear as a mass of finger-sized ridges separated by cracks. These ridges make up the cerebral cortex, and from the top no other structures can be seen. The cerebral cortex in humans is so massive it completely covers the midbrain and hindbrain. Although the cerebral cortex is the most prominent part of the human brain, it is only one of many structures that make up the forebrain. Buried inside the cerebral cortex are groups of cell bodies that comprise the **amygdala, hippocampus, nucleus accumbens, striatum, thalamus,** and other **nuclei.** These structures will be mentioned in subsequent chapters because the midbrain works with them to produce behavior. A more complete understanding of these structures can be found in other books in this series (i.e., *The Forebrain*; *Learning and Memory*).

Remove the brain from the skull and the hindbrain becomes visible protruding down from the middle of the brain. Three parts of the hindbrain are evident from this view—the **pons, medulla oblongata,** and **cerebellum** (Figure 1.1). The pons is a bulbous structure at the top and front of the hindbrain. The medulla oblongata extends from the pons and becomes continuous with the spinal cord as it descends. The cerebellum is attached to the back of the pons by large fiber bundles on each side. Many other structures can be found inside the pons, medulla oblongata, and cerebellum (see *The Hindbrain* book in this series).

THE MIDBRAIN

The midbrain is hidden by the forebrain and the hindbrain. A glimpse of the midbrain is possible only by flipping the brain upside down and looking at the bottom. From this angle, a small part of the midbrain is visible directly in the middle of the brain. It is surrounded by the temporal lobes of the cerebral cor-

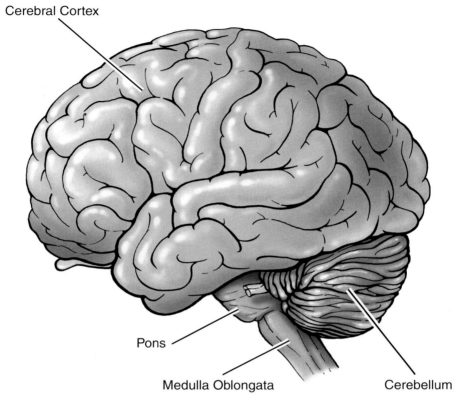

Cerebral Cortex

Pons

Medulla Oblongata

Cerebellum

Figure 1.1 The midbrain is hidden on a lateral view of the brain. The cerebral cortex is extremely large in the human brain and covers most of the other structures. Hindbrain structures such as the pons, medulla oblongata, and cerebellum extend from the bottom of the brain. The midbrain is located just above the pons.

tex on the right and left, the pons on the posterior side, and the hypothalamus on the anterior side (Figure 1.2). A more complete view of the midbrain is possible only by slicing through the brain and peeking inside.

There are several ways the brain can be cut. The view that best shows the relationship of the midbrain to other structures is made possible by cutting the brain down the middle into equal right and left halves (Figure 1.3). This **midsagittal** cut reveals a small bundle of tissue connecting the huge forebrain on top and

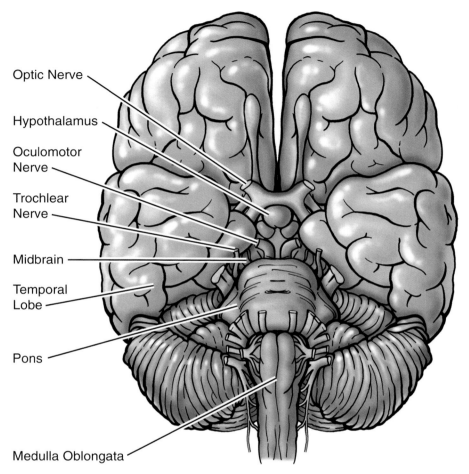

Optic Nerve

Hypothalamus

Oculomotor Nerve

Trochlear Nerve

Midbrain

Temporal Lobe

Pons

Medulla Oblongata

Figure 1.2 A view of the bottom, or ventral, side of the brain reveals a small piece of the midbrain. The midbrain is located in the center stuffed between the pons and hypothalamus and covered by the temporal lobes of the cerebral cortex. Two small nerves can be seen emerging from the midbrain—the oculomotor nerve in the middle and the trochlear nerve at the edge of the midbrain.

the elongated hindbrain below. The midbrain is the only tissue connecting the forebrain and hindbrain. All of the information entering the forebrain except sight and smell must pass through the midbrain. Likewise, forebrain control of the body is made possible by fibers passing through the midbrain. These path-

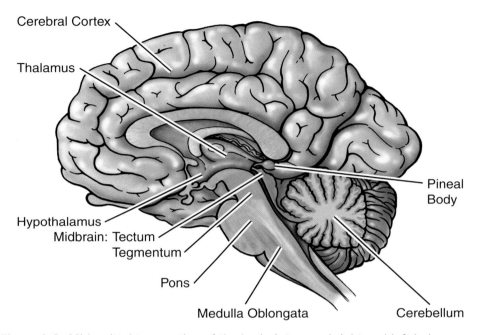

Figure 1.3 Midsagittal transection of the brain into equal right and left halves provides the best opportunity to see the midbrain in relation to other brain structures. The massive forebrain includes all the tissue above and lateral to the midbrain. The pons, medulla oblongata, and cerebellum are found below the midbrain. The fluid-filled cerebral aqueduct provides a clear demarcation of the two major sections of the midbrain, the tectum and tegmentum.

ways are best seen from inside the midbrain (Chapter 8). Although a midsagittal cut reveals very few structures, it does expose the **cerebral aqueduct**. From this view the cerebral aqueduct separates the midbrain into a top part called the tectum and a bottom part called the tegmentum.

Most structures are hidden inside the midbrain. The best way to view these structures is to lay the brain stem flat and slice it into round disks as if cutting a cucumber. These are called **coronal sections**. The structures revealed will depend on whether the cut is close to the thalamus (anterior midbrain) or the pons (posterior midbrain).

The structures that make up the midbrain range from tiny groups of cells such as the **oculomotor** and **trochlear** nuclei that control eye movements (Chapter 5) to large structures such as the **periaqueductal gray** (Chapter 6) that traverse the entire length of the midbrain. Some structures like the **superior** (Chapter 5) and **inferior colliculi** (Chapter 4) protrude from the midbrain, forming two round mounds on the back. Other structures, such as the **red nucleus**, stand out because of their round shape and pinkish color (Chapter 3). Color also distinguishes the **substantia nigra**. This "black substance" is embedded among the white fibers near the bottom of the midbrain (Chapter 3). The substantia nigra and **ventral tegmental** area (Chapter 7) are distinctive in that they are two of the primary sources of the neurotransmitter **dopamine** in the brain.

A coronal section through the midbrain reveals the same structures on both the right and left sides (Figure 1.4). The two mounds at the top of the anterior midbrain are the right and left superior colliculi. Three prominent structures are located at the bottom of the midbrain. The **red nucleus** and **ventral tegmental area** reside near the midline, and the substantia nigra is located more laterally. The cerebral aqueduct, seen along the midline, is a fluid-filled cavity that is part of a canal system running from the cerebral cortex to the spinal cord. The donut-shaped structure surrounding the aqueduct is called the periaqueductal gray. Embedded in the bottom of the **periaqueductal gray** are the oculomotor and trochlear nuclei. Although small, these two nuclei control a complex series of muscles that move the eye (Chapter 5).

Most of the structures mentioned above cannot be seen in a coronal section through the posterior midbrain. The superior colliculi are replaced by two other round mounds at the top called the inferior colliculi. The cerebral aqueduct eventually opens up into the fourth ventricle that runs above the pons and medulla. The periaqueductal gray is still present, but as the

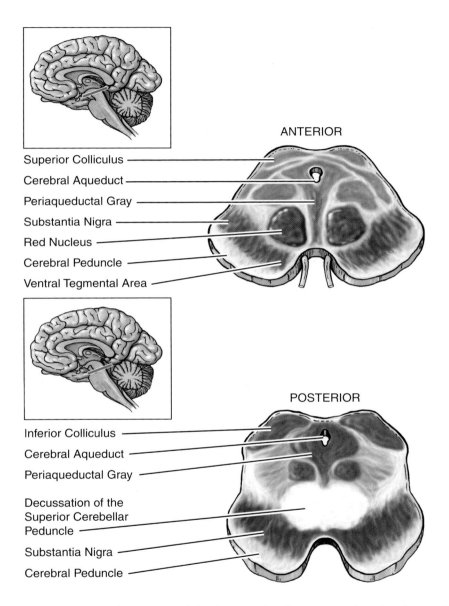

ANTERIOR

Superior Colliculus

Cerebral Aqueduct

Periaqueductal Gray

Substantia Nigra

Red Nucleus

Cerebral Peduncle

Ventral Tegmental Area

POSTERIOR

Inferior Colliculus

Cerebral Aqueduct

Periaqueductal Gray

Decussation of the
Superior Cerebellar
Peduncle

Substantia Nigra

Cerebral Peduncle

Figure 1.4 A slice through the midbrain reveals all of the major structures. The anterior midbrain is dominated by the superior colliculus at the top and the red nucleus toward the bottom. These structures are replaced in the posterior midbrain by the inferior colliculus and the decussation of the superior cerebellar peduncle. The periaqueductal gray, substantia nigra, and cerebral peduncle are present throughout the anterior/posterior extent of the midbrain.

aqueduct expands, the top of the periaqueductal gray shrinks. Structures at the bottom of the brain such as the substantia nigra and ventral tegmental area are much smaller or, in the case of the red nucleus, disappear completely. Huge fiber bundles called the crux cerebri make up most of the bottom of the midbrain. In fact, much of the space outside the well-defined borders of the structures described above consists of the **mesencephalic reticular formation** and various fibers carrying messages from one place to another.

NEURONS

Pictures of the brain make it look like a solid structure. Microscopic analysis reveals that the brain is composed of two broad classes of cells and a lot of empty space. **Neurons** are a type of cell involved in transmitting messages from one area to another. **Glia**, which maintain and support neurons, make up the rest of the brain. Although often overlooked, the brain could not function without glia. There are approximately 100 billion neurons in the brain and glia appear to be even more numerous. (See the book *Cells of the Nervous System.*)

Although there are many different types of neurons (e.g., **Purkinje cells, motoneurons**), the basic organization of cell body, **dendrite**, and **axon** is the same. The cell body is a round or star-shaped structure involved in maintaining normal cell functions. In particular, the cell body contains DNA and organelles (or body parts within a cell) that allow proteins to be made. Proteins are involved in all aspects of neuronal functioning. Dendrites are short branching structures extending from the cell body. Dendrites are designed to receive and transmit information to the cell body. The axon projects from the cell body so that information can be transmitted to other neurons or targets (i.e., muscles, glands) (Figure 1.5). Axons are often insulated with what is called a myelin sheath. Myelin gives axons a white appearance and allows messages to be transmitted rapidly over long distances.

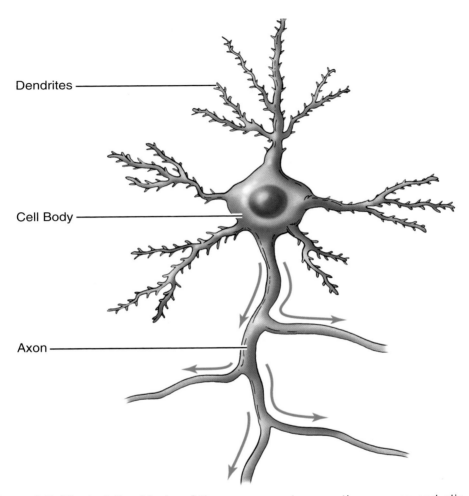

Dendrites

Cell Body

Axon

Figure 1.5 The building blocks of the nervous system are the neurons and glia. Neurons have three distinct parts, the dendrite, cell body, and axon, which allow them to receive and send messages. Messages typically arrive on the dendrites, are collected in the cell body, and are transmitted to distant locations by the axon. The cell body also contains DNA and organelles that maintain the healthy functioning of the neuron.

A slice through the brain will reveal gray and white regions. The gray regions are clusters of cell bodies. A group of neurons is referred to as a **nucleus** (e.g., red nucleus). The axons emanating from these neurons tend to travel through the brain together. These bundles of axons are called **tracts** (e.g., **corti-cospinal tract**). Neuroscientists have labeled hundreds of structures in the brain (see "The Birth of Neuroscience" box) in much the same way geographers label cities and roads. A city is like a nucleus and the roads connecting cities are like axon tracts.

The Birth of Neuroscience

Everyone knows that the brain is the organ that allows us to feel, think, and move. Two thousand years ago, this was not known and was disputed by one of the greatest thinkers of all time. Aristotle argued that intellect resided in the heart, and the brain was a radiator used to cool the blood. Aristotle believed that humans are rational beings because the large human brain facilitates cooling the blood, thus calming the heart. Although Aristotle's conception of the brain is logical, it is wrong. Aristotle's mistake raises an important question: How does one determine the function of the brain? There are many techniques available to humans today that were not available 2,000 or even 100 years ago. Galen (A.D. 130–200), a Roman physician for gladiators, shifted focus from the heart to the brain by dissecting the brains of animals and observing the effects of brain damage on gladiator behavior. Anatomical and lesion studies are useful techniques still in use today. However, these techniques were insufficient to launch the field of neuroscience. In the 19th century, several key advances provided the foundation to begin to understand the nervous system. Luigi Galvani discovered that the nervous system used electricity to transmit messages. Paul Broca demonstrated that specific functions such as language are localized to specific brain structures. Theodor Schwann identified neurons as the units that make up the nervous system. Once started, neuroscience showed incredible growth during the 20th century—a trend that is sure to continue.

■ **Learn more about the history of neuroscience** Search the Internet for *neuroscience history*.

The midbrain is full of axons (Chapter 8). These axons carry messages from the brain to the body and from the body to the brain. Axons also transmit information from one part of the midbrain to another and commonly connect a structure on one side with the identical structure on the opposite side. These connections allow the right side of the body to know what the left side is doing. The tiny axons that allow communication within a nucleus are much too small to see without the help of a powerful microscope.

COMMUNICATION

The primary function of a neuron is to transmit a message from one place to another. Two distinct processes are necessary for neuronal communication. A neuron must move the message from the dendrites and cell body to the tip of the axon, and then transmit that message to another neuron or suitable target (e.g., muscle, gland). Transmission of messages within a neuron is electrical and transmission between neurons is chemical.

An electrical signal is produced in neurons in your skin when someone touches you. This electrical message is transmitted the entire length of the neuron until it reaches the tip of the axon, called the terminal button. Electricity causes the terminal button to release a chemical called a **neurotransmitter**. There are many different types of neurotransmitters (e.g., dopamine, serotonin, glutamate, GABA, enkephalin). The neurotransmitter floats across a tiny gap called a synapse and binds to a **receptor** on another neuron. A receptor is a uniquely shaped protein that has a docking site for a particular type of neurotransmitter. Channels on the neuron open or close when the neurotransmitter binds to the receptor, causing changes in the electrical signal in the neuron. These changes can excite or inhibit a neuron. If the change is excitatory, then an electrical signal is more likely to occur and be transmitted down the axon of the neuron, causing the neurotransmitter to be released. This process is replicated from neuron to neuron carrying messages throughout the nervous system.

Given that there are 100 billion neurons in the brain, the brain is constantly sending messages. An understanding of the electrical and chemical signaling of the brain is important for two reasons. First, much of what is known about the function of the brain has been discovered by artificially stimulating neurons or injecting substances that mimic neurotransmitters. Throughout this book, the function of structures will be described in terms of the effects of electrical or chemical activation. The second reason understanding communication is important is that connections between structures imply a functional relationship. Most of the descriptions of nuclei in this book will include a discussion of the connections with other structures. These connections can be excitatory or inhibitory and merely indicate that two structures can communicate.

■ **Learn more about neural communication** Search the Internet for *neurotransmitter, synaptic transmission,* and *action potential.*

SUMMARY

The goal of this chapter was to introduce you to the midbrain. You should have an overview of the relationship of the midbrain to the rest of the brain, a sense of the different structures within the midbrain, and an understanding of how neurons in the midbrain and elsewhere communicate. The remaining chapters will describe the contribution of midbrain structures to a wide range of behaviors. The complexity of these behaviors will amaze you, given that most of what the midbrain does is below conscious awareness. Enjoy your journey through the midbrain.

2 | Comparative Neuroanatomy: Is Bigger Better?

If you were to create a new superhero, you might name it *The Animal. The Animal* has many superpowers. It can see a mouse in the grass from a distance of six football fields; identify every person in your school using its sense of smell; detect the presence of other animals by the electric discharges in their muscles; sleep with half the brain at a time so it is always alert; run as fast as the cars on the freeway; track fleeing animals in complete darkness using sound; and run across the thinnest of tightropes without falling. Although *The Animal* would fit in well with the cast of *The Incredibles*, this superhero is not a computer-generated comic. *The Animal* is a composite of some of the amazing traits found in animals living on this planet. The vision of a hawk is so acute that it can see a mouse 600 meters (550 yards) away. A dog can track a criminal by the smell of his shirt. Sturgeon use electroreception to detect animals hidden in river mud. A dolphin remains alert and swimming while half its brain sleeps at a time. The cheetah can sprint to speeds of 70 mph (112 km/hr). A bat's hearing is so acute that it can locate and catch insects in complete darkness. Squirrels easily scamper along wires and branches without falling. These extraordinary talents make humans seem ordinary—not the top of the animal kingdom as we tend to view ourselves. The ability of humans to think and solve problems also is an extraordinary talent, but this talent is no more advanced than the vision of a hawk or a dog's sense of smell.

The point is that every animal has special skills that allow it to succeed in a particular environment. These behavioral adaptations are matched by adaptations in both the body and brain. For example, both the ears and a midbrain structure called the inferior colliculus (see Chapter 4) are quite large in bats. These adaptations allow bats to know the distance and direction of flight of a tiny insect by listening to echoes of sound waves bouncing off the bug. This chapter examines some of the variations in the midbrain of different animals that allow these different skills. This field of research, called comparative neuroanatomy, provides fascinating insights into the relationship between neural structures and behavior.

RELATIVE VS. ABSOLUTE SIZE

As mentioned in Chapter 1, the midbrain is a small structure stuck between the hindbrain and forebrain. The degree to which the midbrain influences behavior in different species depends on the size of the midbrain relative to the rest of the brain. The relative size of the midbrain varies drastically across species. The unusually large cerebral cortex in humans results in a relatively small midbrain. Animals with a smaller cerebral cortex, such as a shark, have a relatively large midbrain. This difference does not mean that humans are superior to sharks, just that the forebrain plays a more important role in directing human behavior and the midbrain plays a more important role in directing shark behavior. Your forebrain allows for complex thoughts, so you assume you are more advanced than a shark, but that myth is quickly debunked when you find yourself swimming in the ocean where the shark's midbrain is more than a match for your forebrain. The success of a species is determined by how well it

Table 2.1 Brain-to-Body Size Ratios

	BODY WEIGHT	BRAIN WEIGHT	BRAIN/BODY RATIO
Dolphin	170 kg	~1500–1600 g	0.9%
Human	65 kg	1400 g	2.2%
Chimpanzee	60 kg	420 g	0.7%
Alligator	220 kg	8.4 g	0.004%
Rat	0.4 kg	2 g	0.5%

Source: Neuroscience for Kids. *http://faculty.washington.edu/chudler/facts.html*

is adapted to its environment, not how big its brain is. The midbrain of the shark allows it to be very successful in its environment, just like the cerebral cortex allows you to be successful in your environment.

Comparison of brain size reveals that the human brain (1400 g, 3.1 pounds) is much larger than a great white shark's brain (34 g, 1.2 ounces), which in turn, is larger than a cat's brain (30 g, 1.1 ounces). Such comparisons reveal very little about animals other than to make humans feel superior (just to keep you humble, the brain of a dolphin is significantly larger than that of a human). One reason such comparisons are not useful is that brain size is related to body size. Large animals tend to have large brains. Large people tend to have larger brains than smaller people. Thus, any comparison of brain size must take into account the size of the animal. Comparison of relative brain size is accomplished by dividing brain weight by body weight. Table 2.1 shows the relative brain weight of a number of animals. As you can see by comparing the alligator and rat, relative brain size has as much to do with a large body as with a small brain.

Comparing the size of the midbrain of different animals also is meaningless without adjusting for the relative size of the brain. When this adjustment is made, humans have an extremely small midbrain compared to most other animals. Of course, the reason for the relatively small size of the midbrain in humans is that the forebrain is exceptionally large. This large forebrain has taken over and enhanced many of the functions of the midbrain. For example, a bird has a relatively large midbrain and exceptional vision. Although visual acuity is better in hawks compared to humans, the development of visual centers in the cerebral cortex of humans allows conscious awareness of what is seen—a skill probably limited to primates. Comparison of the relative size of the midbrain in a variety of species suggests that the midbrain is much more important in mediating behavior in most animals compared to humans. That is, the midbrain plays a much greater role in converting input to behavior in most animals compared to humans, in which the cerebral cortex regulates much of the output of the midbrain. Figure 2.1 shows the relative size of the midbrain in a variety of species. Of course, the relative size of the cerebral cortex is greater in humans than in other animals. The key factor that determines the size of the midbrain is the size of the individual structures within it. Although comparison of overall brain size reveals very little, comparison of the size of specific structures in the brain is important in that such comparisons reveal links between brain structure and function.

MIDBRAIN STRUCTURES

Structures in the midbrain are extremely well conserved across species. The term "conserved" in comparative anatomy means that the same structure is present across a wide range of species. Through the course of evolution, traits are lost or acquired as animals adapt to particular environments. This is true with humans, as is evident with the lightening of skin color as humans migrated to northern climates where the shorter days make it difficult to absorb vitamin D from sunlight. Brain structures also have been modified, added, and lost as animals have

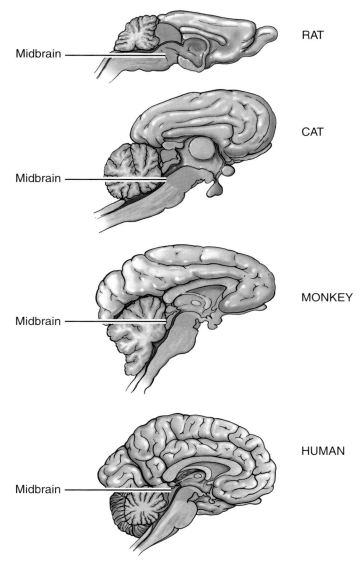

Figure 2.1 A midsagittal section through the brains of four animals shows the relative size of the midbrain compared to the overall size of the brain. The midbrain makes up a relatively large part of the midbrain in the rat and cat. The relative size of the midbrain is much smaller in the monkey and human because the cerebral cortex is quite large. All brains are drawn the same size even though the rat brain (2 g; 0.7 ounces) is significantly smaller than the human brain (1400 g; 3.1 pounds).

evolved. Despite the drastic changes in body types (compare birds and fish), the same midbrain structures are found in nearly all vertebrates. The primary difference between animals is the size and location of these midbrain structures. For example, the **optic tectum**, **torus semicircularis**, and red nucleus are clearly seen when looking at a cross section through the midbrain of a fish, shark, frog, lizard, and bird (Figure 2.2). Given that each of these animals is quite different, the size and shape of these structures also are quite different. In particular, look at the difference in size and location of the red nucleus in these animals. The amazing thing is that this structure exists in such a wide range of animals.

These structures also are present in the human brain even though the names of the optic tectum and torus semicircularis have been changed to superior colliculus and inferior colliculus, respectively (Figure 2.3). The relative sizes of the human superior and inferior colliculi are significantly smaller than the optic tectum and torus semicircularis in most other animals. This difference is related to the growth of the forebrain in humans which has assumed control of many of the functions mediated by these structures. For example, the optic tectum, which is involved in vision, is extremely large in animals with exceptional vision, such as birds (see Figure 2.3). Although the superior colliculus also contributes to vision in humans (see Chapter 5), human vision is not as acute as that of a bird. Much of human vision is coded by neurons in the **occipital cortex** of the forebrain.

Another difference is that the torus semicircularis can function to detect electrical currents or to detect sound waves (see "Electroreception" box). The relatively small size of the torus semicircularis in animals able to detect electric currents suggests that processing such information is relatively simple. Animals lacking the ability to detect electric currents tend to have a large torus semicircularis or inferior colliculus as in the case of humans. As will become evident in Chapter 4, coding auditory

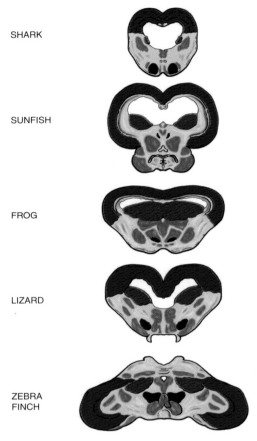

SHARK

SUNFISH

FROG

LIZARD

ZEBRA
FINCH

Figure 2.2 A coronal section through the midbrain allows the interior structures to be seen. Although the size, shape, and location of these structures vary from animal to animal, the same structures can be found despite the extreme differences in the behavior of sharks, fishes, frogs, lizards, and birds. These figures highlight three structures. The red nucleus (red color) varies in size and shape, but tends to be located at the bottom of the midbrain in all animals. The optic tectum (green color) is involved in vision and is relatively large in all of these animals. One major change is that the optic tectum has moved to a lateral position in the zebra finch compared to a location at the top of the midbrain in most animals. The toris semicircularis (blue color) contributes to electroreception in sharks and hearing in land animals. The relatively small size of the toris semicircularis in sharks suggests that electroreception requires less processing power than that required for hearing. The large dark region in the center is the cerebral aqueduct. This canal varies drastically in size and shape. All brains have been adjusted in size for comparison purposes.

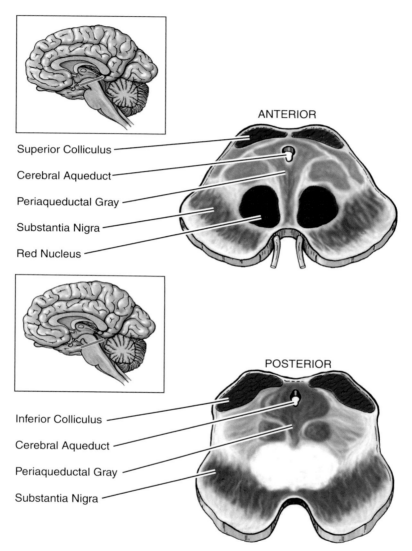

Superior Colliculus

Cerebral Aqueduct

Periaqueductal Gray

Substantia Nigra

Red Nucleus

ANTERIOR

POSTERIOR

Inferior Colliculus

Cerebral Aqueduct

Periaqueductal Gray

Substantia Nigra

Figure 2.3 The human midbrain contains the same structures as in the other vertebrates shown in Figure 2.2. The primary difference is that the optic tectum and toris semicircularis have been renamed as the superior and inferior colliculi in humans. In addition, the inferior colliculus (blue color) has moved to a position at the top border of the midbrain behind the superior colliculus (green color) as opposed to a position below the aqueduct in most other animals. The red nucleus (red color) is quite large in the human midbrain, but its position at the bottom of the midbrain is consistent with other animals.

information is quite complex. One other difference is that the inferior colliculus is located behind the superior colliculus in humans as opposed to below the optic tectum in most other animals.

Electroreception

Ask someone to name all of the sensory systems and most will name five—vision, audition, touch, taste, and smell. No one will include electroreception because this sensory system does not exist in humans. Electroreception is the ability to detect small differences in electric voltages. Given that electric currents can only be conducted through an appropriate medium (e.g., metal, water), electroreception is limited to aquatic animals. This includes such common animals as the catfish and shark, and such odd animals as the platypus. All of these animals have special receptors, typically located on their head and snout, which are activated by a shift in voltage. The ability to detect changes in electric fields is useful in capturing prey, finding mates, and navigating through the ocean. Sharks can detect and capture flounder hidden in the sand by the electric field emanating from the flounder. Sharks also navigate the ocean using electroreception to detect variations in the earth's magnetic field (the movement of water currents through a magnetic field creates a weak electric field). As the shark moves through these electric fields, sensory receptors in the snout transmit messages to the torus semicircularis in the midbrain which, in turn, influences the shark's movement. The torus semicircularis also is used to code sound in land animals. Electroreception does not exist in land animals so the torus semicircularis, or inferior colliculus as it is called in humans, is primarily auditory in function (Chapter 4).

■ **Learn more about vertebrate neuroanatomy** Search the Internet for *brain evolution* and *comparative neuroanatomy.*

SUMMARY

An important lesson from this chapter is that the size of the brain is not a measure of an animal's success. The behavior and bodies of animals vary greatly. Thus, it is not surprising that the brain also varies. The size of particular brain structures corresponds with these behavioral adaptations. The second lesson is that despite the incredible range of behaviors and body adaptations, the structures of the brain are remarkably well conserved. The size and shape of brain structures change, but the structures themselves are evident in animals as different as fish, birds, and humans.

3 | Movement: Two Colorful Nuclei

An ambulance pulls up to the hospital and unloads. The gurney is lowered from the vehicle and wheeled into the emergency room. The patient has no apparent injury and lies completely motionless except for movement of the eyes. A few minutes later another "frozen" person is dropped off. The patients remain rigid as they are transferred to beds. The doctors converge on these patients asking them questions, but neither patient can move and thus cannot talk. The doctors are puzzled because these people appear to be 20 years old, but their symptoms resemble that of a 70-year-old with Parkinson's disease. Parkinson's disease is a movement disorder that begins with difficulty initiating movements and progresses to complete paralysis. Parkinson's disease rarely occurs in someone under 40 years of age yet within a few days, six other young people are brought to hospitals in the area with this same Parkinson's-like immobility. Given these symptoms, the doctors decide to inject levodopa—a treatment that temporarily restores movement to Parkinson's patients. Within minutes, movement is restored, and for the first time the doctors get answers to their questions. All of the patients had taken a heroin-like drug prior to becoming immobile. Scientists analyze the substance and find a synthetic drug called MPPP. MPPP is designed to produce effects similar to heroin. The scientists also find a related chemical called MPTP that was accidentally produced by the novice chemist trying to make MPPP. When injected into laboratory animals, MPTP selectively kills neurons in a midbrain structure called the substantia nigra—the same neurons that die in Parkinson's patients. All of these young people had injected MPTP and now they have an advanced and irreversible form of Parkinson's disease. This happened in the summer of 1982, and these people remain immobile. This chapter will describe the substantia nigra and other midbrain structures involved in movement.

THE SUBSTANTIA NIGRA

The story above is remarkable because MPTP is very selective in that it only kills neurons in the substantia nigra. The death of these neurons is sufficient to prevent all voluntary movements. Other types of movement such as reflexes and learned patterns are mediated by other parts of the nervous system. These types of movements remain intact after damage to the substantia nigra. For example, reflexes such as blinking when dust blows into your eye, or kicking your leg when a physician taps the patella tendon are not altered. Learned automatic movements, such as walking or playing the piano, do not require the substantia nigra except to initiate the movement (a Parkinson's patient can walk if there is a way to get started). The substantia nigra is a key structure in translating the thought "I want some ice cream" into movements such as standing, walking, opening the freezer, and scooping ice cream. Studies examining people who have Parkinson's disease have revealed the important role the substantia nigra plays in initiating movements (see "Parkinson's Disease" box).

The substantia nigra (Latin for black substance) is a large band of dark neurons near the bottom of the midbrain (Figure

3.1). The darkness of these neurons is offset by the white color of the fibers that pass both above and below. On closer examination, two parts of the substantia nigra can be distinguished. The top part is called the substantia nigra pars compacta and the bottom part is called the substantia nigra pars reticulata. The pars compacta neurons are one of the few brain structures that produce the neurotransmitter **dopamine**. Dopamine has

Parkinson's Disease

Neurons in the brain die every day. Given that there are approximately 100 billion neurons in your brain, you could lose 200,000 neurons a day for life and still have over 92 billion remaining when you turn 100 years old. However, if 80% of the neurons in the substantia nigra die, you will join the 1.5 million Americans with Parkinson's disease (60,000 new cases each year). Parkinson's disease is a movement disorder characterized by uncontrolled shaking of the limbs, extremely slow movements (it can take hours to shower and dress), and rigidity. The symptoms get progressively worse until the person is completely immobile except for the shaking. Although the symptoms can be reduced by drugs that increase dopamine levels in the brain or by altering the activity of a structure called the *globus pallidus* through electrical stimulation or brain lesions, currently there is no cure (brain lesions can increase neural activity by removing inhibitory inputs). In addition, there is no way to predict who will get Parkinson's disease, although environmental toxins and genetic factors have been implicated in some cases. Scientists hope that replacing dopamine-containing cells in the brain may one day lead to a cure, but both political (i.e., opposition to stem cell research) and technical problems are major obstacles.

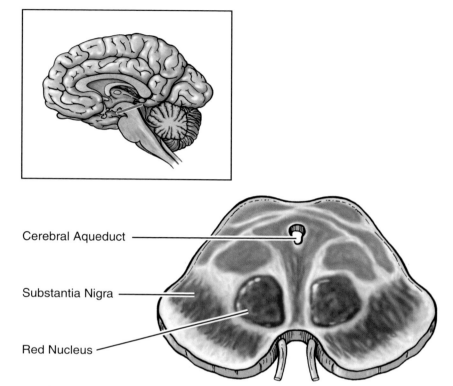

Figure 3.1 Coronal section through the midbrain reveals two colorful and prominent motor nuclei—the substantia nigra and the red nucleus. The substantia nigra has a black appearance because these neurons contain a dark melanin-like pigment. Neurons in the substantia nigra also contain the neurotransmitter dopamine. The red nucleus has a pink appearance because of a thick network of blood vessels.

been identified as a key neurotransmitter in a number of neurological disorders (see "Dopamine-Related Disorders" box) and plays an important role in signaling reward (see Chapter 7). It is the death of these dopamine-containing neurons that causes Parkinson's disease.

BASAL GANGLIA

Although the substantia nigra is located in the midbrain, it is closely linked with a group of structures in the forebrain called the basal ganglia. The structures in the basal ganglia (i.e., the striatum, **globus pallidus**, and parts of the thalamus) provide the circuitry for voluntary movement. Given that all of these struc-

Dopamine-Related Disorders

Dopamine is a neurotransmitter that is produced by neurons in only a few brain regions. Two of these, the substantia nigra and the ventral tegmental area (see Chapter 7), are located in the midbrain. Despite its limited distribution, dopamine is very important to the normal functioning of the brain. The box called "Parkinson's Disease" describes how the loss of dopamine-containing neurons in the substantia nigra leads to Parkinson's disease. In contrast, too much dopamine can lead to Tourette's syndrome, a disorder characterized by uncontrolled movements. These movements can be as common as a face twitch or as embarrassing as uncontrolled shouting and swearing. Dopamine also has been linked to schizophrenia. Schizophrenia is a complex and fascinating disorder characterized by disruption of normal thinking. This can include hallucinations (e.g., hearing voices), disorganized thinking, and lack of appropriate emotions. Although there are no similarities in the symptoms or incidence of Tourette's syndrome and schizophrenia, both disorders can be treated by blocking the action of dopamine. Altering dopamine levels also is used to treat attention deficit hyperactivity disorder (ADHD). However, in this case, treatments such as taking the drug Ritalin® increase dopamine levels. The key to understanding the role of dopamine in these disorders is knowing the various neural circuits that dopamine influences.

■ **Learn more about dopamine-related movement disorders** Search the Internet for *dopamine movement* or the name of a specific disorder.

tures are interconnected, damage to any one results in a movement disorder. Neurons in the substantia nigra project to the striatum. The striatum sends a message back to the substantia nigra as well as to the globus pallidus. Both the globus pallidus and substantia nigra pars reticulata project to the thalamus (Figure 3.2). The thalamus weighs these inputs and sends a message to the cerebral cortex to initiate voluntary movements.

VOLUNTARY MOVEMENT CIRCUIT

Sensory systems are closely linked to brain centers involved in movement. This allows you to respond to things you see, hear, touch, and smell. For example, the smell of cookies baking will cause you to stand up and walk into the kitchen where you may find freshly baked cookies. The sight and smell of these cookies activate brain centers that temporarily transform you into the Cookie Monster—that is, you want to grab and eat the cookies. The process of grabbing a cookie seems simple, but it involves the coordination of many brain regions and many muscles. The brain regions that process sensory information (e.g., smell, vision) send messages to the premotor cortex describing where the cookie is located. The premotor cortex prepares a plan to activate the muscles necessary to grab the cookie. This involves coordinating muscles in the legs, back, shoulder, arm, and hand. Once the neurons that cause these muscles to move are prepared, the basal ganglia send a message to the premotor cortex initiating the motor plan. This plan is forwarded to the primary motor cortex which activates motoneurons in the spinal cord. Each motoneuron causes fibers in a specific muscle to contract. Contraction of muscles causes bones to move allowing you to reach and grab the cookie. As you can see, even seemingly simple movements are quite complex.

If you've ever accidentally knocked over a glass of milk or tripped over a step, you know that the premotor cortex does not always outline an accurate plan. Coordination of all the neurons

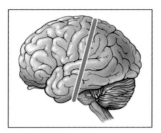

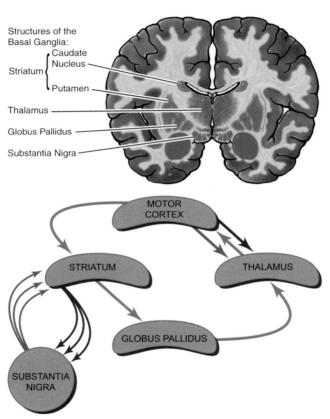

Figure 3.2 The basal ganglia is a network of structures underlying the production of voluntary movements. These structures include the substantia nigra, which sends and receives messages to the striatum in the forebrain. The striatum transmits information to the globus pallidus, which in turn transmits the message to the thalamus. The thalamus signals the motor cortex to trigger movements. A carefully placed coronal section through the brain reveals all of these structures (top). The connections between these structures are shown schematically at the bottom of this illustration.

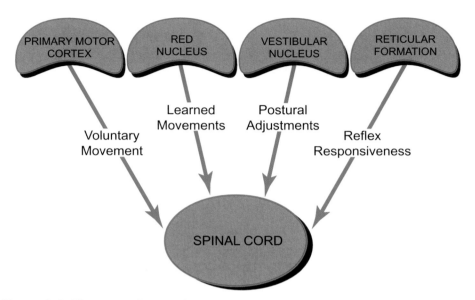

Figure 3.3 There are four major descending pathways that control movement. These are the corticospinal, rubrospinal, vestibulospinal, and reticulospinal tracts. Each pathway starts in a different brain structure and has a different function. All four pathways terminate on motoneurons in the spinal cord. These descending pathways also terminate in the brainstem to control the muscles of the head and neck.

and muscles necessary for a precise movement is the result of years of learning. This process is particularly vivid if you've ever watched a baby learn to stand and walk. After much trial and error, the baby's nervous system learns to control and coordinate the muscles necessary to stand and walk. Sensory feedback is very important in this process because it corrects movements as they occur. Four distinct but interconnected motor circuits are necessary for coordinated movements. In addition to the corticospinal tract, which runs from the **primary motor cortex** to the spinal cord and is involved in voluntary movements, the **vestibulospinal**, **reticulospinal**, and **rubrospinal tracts** also contribute to the smooth execution of movements (Figure 3.3). The vestibulospinal tract adjusts posture based on the movement and position of the head. The reticulospinal tract regulates muscle tone and reflex responsiveness. The rubrospinal tract arises from a midbrain structure called the red nucleus and is described below.

■ **Learn more about neural control of movement** Search the Internet for *motor coordination, cerebellum,* and *basal ganglia.*

RED NUCLEUS

Located above the substantia nigra on each side of the brain is the colorful red nucleus. If you are dissecting a freshly cut brain, the actual color is more pink than red, but scientists, not artists, named the structure. The pink color is the result of a thick network of blood vessels in this region. The red nucleus is easy to find in the human brain because of its color and round shape (see Figure 3.1).

The function of the red nucleus matches that of the primary motor cortex in many ways. Both receive input from the **sensorimotor cortex** (this part of the cerebral cortex organizes movements based on sensory system input) and contribute to voluntary movements. The **primary motor cortex** dominates movement in humans. In contrast, the red nucleus makes a greater contribution to voluntary movement in most other animals. Damage to the motor cortex in humans inhibits voluntary movements, but cats suffering the same cortical damage are able to walk by relying on neurons in the red nucleus. In most mammals, birds, and reptiles, the red nucleus appears to coordinate the activity of various muscles for both skilled (grasping) and unskilled (walking) movements.

The red nucleus also appears to contribute to executing learned movements. For example, learning a new dance routine requires the coordination and precise timing of many muscles. The timing for these movements is too quick for conscious control so the red nucleus, through reciprocal connections with the cerebellum, provides unconscious control of the muscles. The more you practice, the more automatic and stable these motor circuits become, making you a better dancer, athlete, or musician. Of course, some people are naturally more coordinated than others. Although coordination is a complex interaction between sensory and **motor systems**, differences in how well the red nucleus and cerebellum function are sure to contribute.

Although each motor pathway has a distinct function, the four motor circuits interact at all levels of the nervous system so movement is well coordinated. The cerebellum appears to be a key structure in coordinating movements within the brain. At the spinal level, approximately half the neurons contribute to movement. Neurons in the spinal cord receive input from the corticospinal, vestibulospinal, reticulospinal, and rubrospinal tracts (Figure 3.4). Additional input comes directly from muscles, tendons, pain fibers, and neurons from other spinal segments. Motoneurons integrate these various inputs before signaling muscles to contract. Without such coordination, the corticospinal tract could tell your muscles to grab a cookie while the learned pattern coming from your rubrospinal tract tries to play the piano. The reticulospinal and vestibulospinal tracts contribute to movement by adjusting muscle tone based on feedback from the muscles and adjusting posture based on movement of the head, respectively.

SUMMARY

Much of the nervous system is devoted to sensory input and motor output. Thus, it is not surprising that the midbrain is packed with motor nuclei. The substantia nigra and red nucleus are the two most prominent midbrain structures involved in movement. The substantia nigra contributes to the initiation of voluntary movements and is of particular interest because of its role in Parkinson's disease. Less is known about the red nucleus

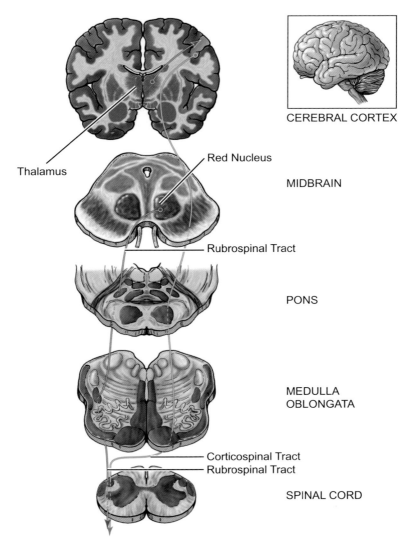

CEREBRAL CORTEX

Thalamus

Red Nucleus

MIDBRAIN

Rubrospinal Tract

PONS

MEDULLA OBLONGATA

Corticospinal Tract
Rubrospinal Tract

SPINAL CORD

Figure 3.4 The corticospinal and rubrospinal tracts contribute to voluntary and learned movements. The corticospinal tract originates from neurons in the motor cortex. Axons from these neurons travel through the forebrain, midbrain, pons, and medulla before crossing to the opposite of the spinal cord and synapsing on motoneurons. The rubrospinal tract originates from neurons in the red nucleus and descends through the pons, medulla, and spinal cord on the opposite side before terminating on motoneurons. The reason these pathways cross to the opposite side remains a mystery.

especially with regard to its function in humans. At the very least, it contributes to learned movements. The midbrain also contains massive fiber systems involved in movement (Chapter 8) in addition to the oculomotor and trochlear nuclei. These midbrain nuclei automatically control eye, head, and body movements and are discussed in more detail in Chapter 5. You do not have to think about these movements because the midbrain takes care of them for you.

4 | The Impressive Inferior Colliculus

A simple experiment that clearly shows the power of the auditory system is to call a friend and simply say, "Hello." If the connection is good and the friend knows you well, then that one word will be all that is needed to identify you. Given that there are hundreds of voices you hear every week, the ability of the auditory system to identify someone from a single word is miraculous. Not only is everyone's voice unique, but the auditory system can distinguish and remember the slight differences in all these voices. This feat becomes even more incredible when you realize that the information transmitted from the phone to your ear is coded by vibrations of the air. Needless to say, the neural processing that allows you to distinguish different sounds is extremely complex. A key player in this processing is a midbrain structure called the inferior colliculus.

WHAT IS SOUND?

All sound is transmitted through vibrations. These vibrations are not evident unless you are watching or touching the speakers on a stereo. Movement of the speaker back and forth creates vibrations in the air. The movement of air near the speaker moves the adjacent air, and in this way, sound travels across a room. (Sound will not travel in a vacuum, such as

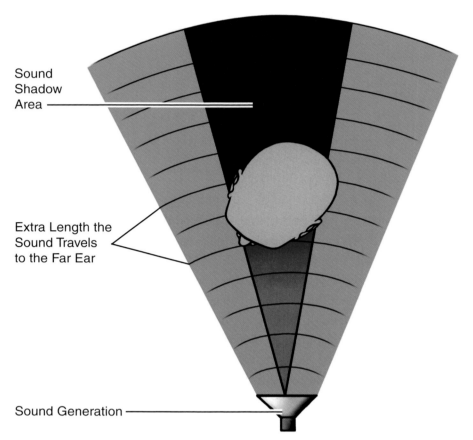

Sound Shadow Area

Extra Length the Sound Travels to the Far Ear

Sound Generation

Figure 4.1 Sounds are generated by vibration of the air. These vibrations are very intense near the source of a sound and become weaker with distance. The sound wave travels in all directions and arrives at your two ears at different times and intensities.

outer space, because there is no air.) The force on the air decreases with the distance the wave travels (Figure 4.1). This phenomenon allows you to whisper to a classmate without the teacher hearing you. Sound waves take time to travel as is evident by sitting in the outfield and seeing a batter hit a baseball. The sound of the bat hitting the ball takes a second or two to reach you. Eventually these vibrations of the air enter your ear, causing your eardrum to vibrate. In contrast, light travels much faster so seeing the ball hit the bat is almost instantaneous. Vibrations of the eardrum are transmitted to the inner ear where specialized neurons convert vibrations into neural activity.

Mechanical vibrations are converted to neural activity inside a spiral-shaped structure called the **cochlea**. The cochlea is a fluid-filled chamber with a flexible **basilar membrane** running through the middle. Vibration of the fluid inside the cochlea causes the basilar membrane to move up and down. Specialized neurons called **hair cells** reside on the basilar membrane. These cells look like they have hair (called stereocilia) sprouting off the top and stuck into an inflexible **tectorial membrane** above. Movement of the basilar membrane causes the stereocilia to bend and neurotransmitter to be released from the hair cells (Figure 4.2).

The hair cells on the basilar membrane are arranged so you can detect the intensity and frequency of sound waves. Intense sound waves are perceived as loud and are caused by strong vibrations of the air. Less intense sound waves are perceived as quiet. As you turn the volume up on a stereo, the movement of the speakers becomes much more evident. The air vibrates at the same frequency, but the force of each wave is greater. The eardrum is deflected more and the hair cells on the basilar membrane are subjected to greater forces. Extremely loud noises (e.g., a jet engine, music at a concert) result in vibrations you can feel pounding against your body. These sound waves are strong enough to permanently bend or break the stereocilia on top of the hair cell. This can lead to ringing in the ears (called tinnitus) or a permanent loss of hearing. Stereocilia do not grow back after they have been broken, so the hair cell can no longer respond to sounds.

Frequency is defined as the number of sound waves occurring each second. Different objects vibrate the air at different rates.

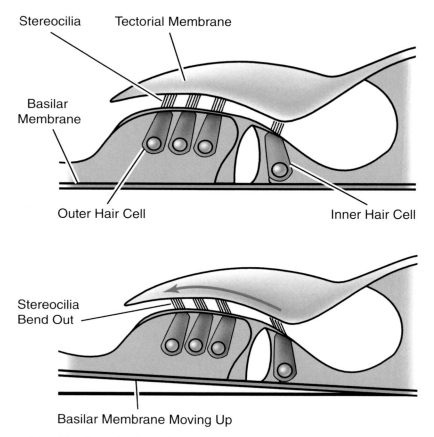

Figure 4.2 Vibrations in the air are converted to mechanical vibrations by the eardrum. The mechanical vibrations cause the basilar membrane in the inner ear to move up and down. Hair cells on the basilar membrane have stereocilia sprouting off the top. The stereocilia are embedded in the rigid tectorial membrane so that movement of the basilar membrane causes the stereocilia to bend. Bending of the stereocilia causes the hair cell to release neurotransmitters onto neurons that make up the auditory nerve. Through this process, the ear transforms vibrations in the air to mechanical vibrations and then to neural activity. Your brain interprets this neural activity as sound.

The long, thick string on a guitar causes fewer vibrations in the air each second than the short, thin string. Your brain perceives these different frequencies as pitch. For example, sound waves arriving 15,000 times a second have a high pitch (e.g., a police siren), whereas sound waves arriving 40 times a second have a low pitch (e.g., a fog horn). The number of air vibrations that occur each second is measured in hertz (Hz). Human perception is limited to sound waves arriving between 20 and 20,000 Hz. Some animals, such as bats, use much higher frequencies (e.g., up to 100,000 Hz). (See "Bat Sonar" box.)

Low- and high-frequency sound waves produce low- and high-pitched sounds by vibrating different parts of the basilar membrane. There are hair cells located across the entire length of the basilar membrane. Each hair cell is activated maximally by a specific frequency. Hair cells located at the beginning of the basilar membrane code high-frequency sounds, and hair cells located at the far end of the basilar membrane code low-frequency sounds. Electrical stimulation of a hair cell located at the end of the basilar membrane will cause you to perceive a low-pitched sound even in the absence of a real sound. The coding of different tones by neurons in different places is called a **tonotopic map**. The auditory system maintains a tonotopic map through all levels of processing, from the hair cells in the inner ear to neurons in the auditory cortex.

Quality of the sound is called timbre and is determined by the number of different and overlapping sound waves. A pure tone, whether it is 20 or 20,000 Hz, travels in a single wave. However, pure tones are very rare. Most sounds are composed of multiple waves arriving at your ear simultaneously. These waves give sounds their complexity and allow different voices to be distinguished. Each person's voice is composed of a unique set of sound waves that can be used to identify people in the same way that fingerprints are unique. Your ear is able to distinguish these different patterns of sound waves by the different patterns of hair cells activated. A sound composed of both low and high frequencies will activate hair cells on two parts of the basilar membrane simultaneously. Given that the patterns of hair cells that can be activated are nearly endless, the variety of different

Bat Sonar

Bats are perhaps the most demonized animals on the planet. Their association with blood-sucking vampires has made them widely feared despite the fact that most bats eat insects. Many bats do not rely on vision to find food because they hunt at night when it is dark. These bats detect and capture insects using echolocation, a type of sonar. Bats emit high-frequency calls that bounce off objects and return to the bat (an echo). The time, strength, and direction of the returning sound wave allow the bat to know the location and direction of flight of an insect. The bat then swoops in and snatches the insect from the air. This amazing ability is made possible by an exceptional auditory system that includes large ears and a well-developed inferior colliculus. A subset of neurons in the inferior colliculus codes the distance to an object by comparing the time between the emitted call and the returning echo. Bats emit very high-frequency sounds (over 40,000 Hz), which is important when trying to gather information from very small insects because the distance between waves is very small (think about 40,000

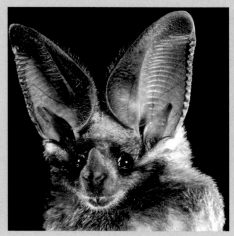

waves per second vs. 20 waves). Given that the human ear can only detect sounds between 20 and 20,000 Hz, the bats flying overhead seem quiet to us. They are actually emitting a continuous barrage of screams—insects beware.

■ **Learn more about bats** Search the Internet for *echolocation* and *bats.*

sounds that can be perceived is also nearly endless (the ability to distinguish different instruments or different voices is a good example).

■ **Learn more about the qualities of sound** Search the Internet for *timbre*, *decibels*, and *sound frequency*.

PATHWAY FROM THE EAR TO THE INFERIOR COLLICULUS

As mentioned above, vibrations in the air are transformed into vibrations of the eardrum that in turn bend the stereocilia on hair cells located on the basilar membrane. Hair cells release a neurotransmitter onto the neurons of the auditory nerve that transmit the message from the inner ear to the **cochlear nucleus** in the medulla oblongata. The cochlear nucleus sends this information to the inferior colliculus and a few other places (e.g., **superior olivary complex**). The inferior colliculus is located in the midbrain. One function of the inferior colliculus is to relay information to the **medial geniculate nucleus** in the thalamus, which in turn transmits information to the auditory cortex located in the temporal lobes of the brain (Figure 4.3). Although information must reach the auditory cortex for conscious awareness of sounds, animals—humans included—can respond to sounds without conscious awareness (you are not conscious while asleep, but sounds are processed and can be incorporated into dreams). All of the processing of auditory information in the inferior colliculus is below conscious awareness.

Auditory information is transformed as it moves through the nervous system from the inner ear to the cerebral cortex. Processing is more complicated in the inferior colliculus than in the cochlear nucleus. The inferior colliculus receives all of the information transmitted from the cochlear nucleus and integrates that information with messages arriving from the nuclei of the **lateral lemniscus**, the **superior olivary complex**, and the

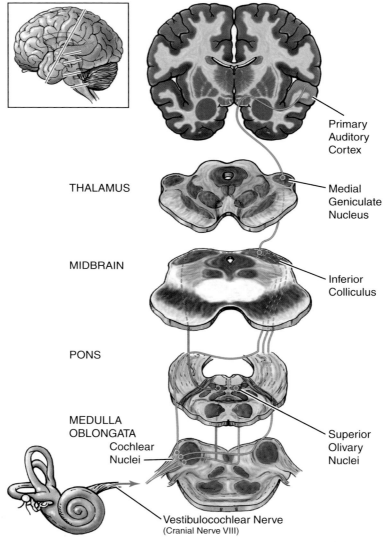

Primary Auditory Cortex

THALAMUS

Medial Geniculate Nucleus

MIDBRAIN

Inferior Colliculus

PONS

MEDULLA OBLONGATA
Cochlear Nuclei

Superior Olivary Nuclei

Vestibulocochlear Nerve
(Cranial Nerve VIII)

Figure 4.3 The pathway from the ear to the auditory cortex where the conscious awareness of sounds occurs is long and complicated. The auditory nerve carries information from hair cells in the inner ear to the cochlear nucleus in the medulla. The cochlear nucleus sends this information to another medullary structure, the superior olivary complex, and via the lateral lemniscus to the inferior colliculus in the midbrain. The superior olivary complex also projects to the inferior colliculus. The inferior colliculus forwards the message to the medial geniculate nucleus in the thalamus and then to the auditory cortex. Somehow, through this process, vibrations of the air are converted to meaningful sounds.

cerebral cortex. Input from the superior olivary complex is particularly interesting because neurons in this structure compare input from the right and left ears so the location of a sound can be determined (see "Localization of Sound"). Thus, the message

Localization of Sound

While walking though a dark forest at night, you hear the crack of a twig to your right. The sound waves from the breaking twig travel in all directions, yet your brain knows exactly where the sound came from. Your brain localizes sounds by comparing the input to your two ears. A sound to the right will hit the right ear earlier and with greater intensity than the left ear. Both ears send this input to a structure called the superior olivary complex, which compares the time and intensity of the signals from the right and left ears. A sound directly in front of you will arrive at both ears simultaneously and activate a different set of neurons in the superior olivary complex than a sound coming from the right or left. The only problem with this system is distinguishing sounds directly in front of and behind you. This problem is solved by a slight turn of the head that will change the distance of the two ears from the sound (cats do this by simply rotating an ear forward or back). Comparing input to the two ears cannot tell you whether a sound came from above or below. The ability to localize sounds up and down depends on the shape of the ear. Neurons in the brain have learned that sounds from above are funneled into the ear differently than sounds coming from below. Changing the shape of your ear by folding the flaps down makes it very difficult to determine whether a sound came from above or below. You can test this by asking a friend to localize the sound of shaking keys while holding their ear flaps down with their eyes closed. This experiment demonstrates the close and important relationship between your body (the shape of your ear) and your brain.

transmitted from the cochlear nucleus to the inferior colliculus is modified by these various other inputs.

■ **Learn more about auditory processing** Search the Internet for *inner ear, auditory pathway,* and *inferior colliculus.*

ANATOMY OF THE INFERIOR COLLICULUS

The word "inferior" suggests that the inferior colliculus is not important. Don't be deceived. Damage to the inferior colliculus will result in complete and profound deafness. The term *inferior* merely refers to location. The inferior colliculus is located behind, or inferior to, the superior colliculus. Despite its name, the inferior colliculus is quite impressive. It is a relatively large structure located at the top and back of the midbrain. It is hidden beneath the cerebral cortex and cerebellum in humans. Removal of these structures reveals the inferior colliculus as a protruding round mound on each side of the midline (Figure 4.4).

Although the inferior colliculus appears as a solid round mound, it has three major subdivisions—the central nucleus, the external cortex, and the dorsal cortex. The central nucleus of the inferior colliculus contains a very precise tonotopic map. As mentioned previously, tonotopic refers to a map of the coding of different tones in adjacent regions. Neurons responding to low-pitched sounds are located near each other and far from neurons responding to high-pitched sounds. This map is consistent with the tonotopic arrangement of the cochlear nucleus that projects to this region of the inferior colliculus.

The subdivision known as the external cortex of the inferior colliculus wraps around the central nucleus. The external cortex is unique in that it receives input from non-auditory structures. This includes input from a medullary structure called the **dorsal column nucleus** that is activated by touch. The external cortex also receives input from the substantia nigra and globus pal-

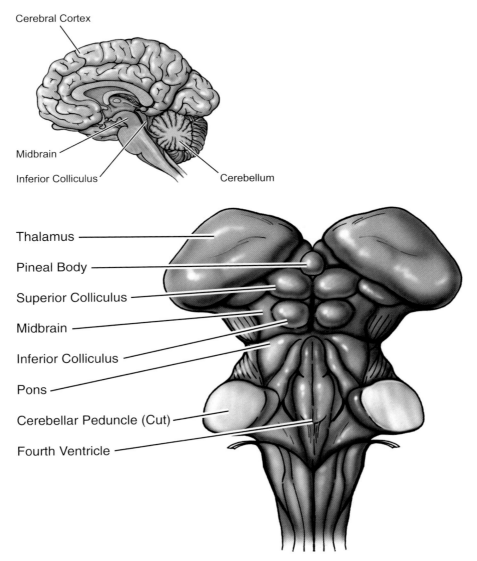

Figure 4.4 In a normal brain, the inferior colliculus is hidden from view by the cerebral cortex and cerebellum. Removal of these two structures allows a clear view of the back side of the midbrain. Two prominent bulges are evident—the superior colliculus in front and the inferior colliculus below. These structures are surrounded by the thalamus in front and the pons behind.

lidus—two structures involved in movement (Chapter 3). Neurons in the external cortex differ from other parts of the inferior colliculus because they respond to both touch and sound.

The third subdivision is called the dorsal cortex of the inferior colliculus. The organization of the neurons in this region is very similar to the neurons in the central nucleus. The primary difference between the two is that the tonotopic organization of neurons in the dorsal cortex is the result of input from the primary auditory cortex, not from lower structures conveying auditory information to the central nucleus of the inferior colliculus.

FUNCTION OF THE INFERIOR COLLICULUS

Learning about brain structures is much more satisfying when a specific function can be assigned to a structure. The excitement inherent in science is trying to understand what a brain structure does and how it does it. There is no textbook or Website that scientists can use to reveal the function of the inferior colliculus. The function of the inferior colliculus remains a puzzle waiting to be solved. It is well known that the inferior colliculus contributes to auditory processing. The problem is that the responses of neurons in the inferior colliculus are similar to the responses of neurons in lower auditory structures such as the superior olivary complex and higher structures like the medial geniculate nucleus and auditory cortex. If neurons in these structures have the same function, then why waste brain space and processing time by duplication? The obvious answer is that these structures do not have the same function. The problem is that our understanding of these structures is incomplete. The process by which a more complete understanding is possible is to examine the current data, devise a hypothesis, and collect data to test the hypothesis.

A few findings provide clues about the possible role of the inferior colliculus in auditory processing. First, the inferior colliculus receives input from all auditory structures located below it. Thus, even though neurons in the inferior colliculus and superior olivary complex may have similar responses, the inferior colliculus integrates input from the superior olivary complex with inputs from other structures. The inferior colliculus also receives input from the auditory cortex, indicating that feedback from higher centers is important. A third clue is that the inferior colliculus receives both excitatory and inhibitory inputs. Given that excitatory inputs are necessary to transmit information, the presence of extensive inhibitory inputs suggests powerful modulation of this excitation.

An obvious assumption is that the processing of sounds becomes increasingly complex as the message moves from the ear to the cerebral cortex. One way to add complexity is to refine the response properties of a neuron. A neuron in the cochlear nucleus responds to a wide range of sounds and, thus, is not very good at distinguishing between these sounds. The cochlear nucleus transmits this same information to the inferior colliculus. However, the inferior colliculus refines this message by eliminating some of the sounds that activated neurons in the cochlear nucleus. For example, a neuron in the cochlear nucleus that responds to any sound wave between 1000 and 2000 Hz will transmit that same information to a neuron in the inferior colliculus. Inhibitory inputs to this neuron in the inferior colliculus will eliminate the response to sound waves below 1300 Hz and above 1700 Hz, leaving a neuron with a more specific response.

Inhibitory inputs also are very useful in signaling the onset and offset of a sound. Activation of a hair cell will cause a continuous barrage of activity in neurons in the auditory nerve and cochlear nucleus. The onset of this input is relayed to the inferior colliculus, where inhibitory inputs will quickly terminate neural activity. Other neurons in the inferior colliculus become active as soon as the barrage of activity stops. Thus, specific neurons in the inferior colliculus code the onset and offset of sounds. Although the function of these responses is not known, a sharp onset and offset would enhance the contrast of new sounds from background noise.

As auditory information makes its way along the pathway from hair cells to auditory cortex, pure tones are transformed into complex sounds and then to words. Although it is not known where these transformations occur, the inferior colliculus plays an important role in this transformation. However, the function of the inferior colliculus is surely greater than merely transforming auditory information and relaying it to the medial geniculate nucleus and auditory cortex. The inferior colliculus has connections to the **pretectal area** and superior colliculus (Chapter 5). These pathways probably allow rapid coordination between auditory and visual stimuli. The delay required to process auditory information in the cortex before coordinating with vision could be quite dangerous when attempting to find prey and avoid predators. Thus, the direct connection from the inferior colliculus to the superior colliculus probably allows you to respond to sounds before you are consciously aware of the sound.

OTHER FUNCTIONS OF THE INFERIOR COLLICULUS

In addition to auditory processing, two interesting findings suggest that the inferior colliculus contributes to defense. First, the inferior colliculus receives input from brain regions involved in touch. Stroking the skin activates neurons in the inferior colliculus. Second, electrical stimulation of the inferior colliculus evokes defensive reactions. Mild activation evokes an alerting response, intermediate activation evokes defensive immobility, and strong activation evokes escape behaviors. Similar responses are produced by activation of the superior colliculus and the periaqueductal gray (Chapter 6). Thus, the inferior colliculus may contribute to a defensive system residing within the midbrain. One possibility is that the inferior and superior colliculi relay information about visual, auditory, and tactile threats to the periaqueductal gray. The periaqueductal gray integrates this information and coordinates an appropriate defensive response.

SUMMARY

Although the precise function of the inferior colliculus remains a mystery for future neuroscientists to solve, the inferior colliculus is a vital part of auditory processing. It codes sounds in a precise tonotopic manner and transmits that information to higher brain centers where conscious awareness and comprehension occur. The inferior colliculus also appears to contribute to defense by directing attention to sounds and touch. It is clear that the inferior colliculus is an impressive structure.

5 | Seeing Without Believing

Professional basketball players are exceptionally talented athletes. Their skills include remarkable quickness, incredible leaping ability, and excellent hand-eye coordination. However, one of the best basketball players of all time, Earvin "Magic" Johnson, was not particularly fast, could not jump very high, and was not a great shooter. The skill that distinguished Earvin from other players, and earned him the nickname "Magic," was an ability to see everyone on the basketball court. He would make seemingly magical passes behind his head to teammates cutting toward the basket. It seemed as though Magic had eyes in the back of his head. His exceptional ability to see his teammates was not because of his eyes, but because of a midbrain structure called the superior colliculus. The superior colliculus coordinates eye and head movements so the location of objects, such as a teammate, can be known. Magic Johnson's superior colliculus functioned so well that he could track all of his teammates and know where they would be in a few seconds. Magic simply delivered the basketball to his teammate when he arrived at that spot. Your superior colliculus tracks the movement of objects in a similar manner, it just doesn't do it as quickly or as well as Magic's superior colliculus. This chapter will describe the superior colliculus and other midbrain structures involved in vision.

TWO VISUAL SYSTEMS

A discussion of the visual system typically focuses on how the brain processes images. Images are identified by their shape, size, and color. The human visual system is so sensitive it can distinguish thousands of colors and an infinite number of shapes. The pathway that codes colors and shapes runs from the retina of the eye to the **lateral geniculate nucleus** in the thalamus to the occipital lobe of the cerebral cortex. This is the system that allows for conscious awareness of the face of a loved one or the beauty of a sunset. However, this is but one part of the visual system. A less well-known part of the visual system allows you to see without conscious awareness. That is, as the title of this chapter hints, you can see without believing you are actually seeing—a phenomenon known as "blind sight" (see "Blind Sight" box).

■ **Learn more about blind sight** Search the Internet for *blind sight* or *unconscious vision.*

The processing of information for the "second" visual system occurs in the midbrain. The midbrain system is comprised of several important structures such as the superior colliculus, **pretectal area**, **interstitial nucleus of Cajal**, and the oculomotor and trochlear nuclei (Figure 5.1). These structures coordinate eye and head movements so objects can be followed. Without this coordination, objects would jitter and jump across your retina, making vision virtually useless. For example, your head moves up and down as you walk. The muscles controlling your eyes compensate for this movement so the world appears steady. Most people are unaware of this system because it happens without conscious awareness. However, damage to this system disrupts vision almost as severely as damage to the conscious visual system because it makes it impossible to hold your gaze on objects as you or the object move. You would not be able to read, drive, or search for a friend in a crowd. Fortunately, there are many structures involved in this system so it is nearly impossible to damage it completely. Each of these midbrain structures contributes to eye movements in a slightly different way and each will be discussed separately.

Blind Sight

The function of a brain structure can be determined by the deficits that occur when the structure is damaged. Damage to midbrain structures such as the superior colliculus or oculomotor nucleus makes it difficult to follow moving objects. In contrast, damage to the primary visual cortex results in blindness. Damage to the visual cortex also reveals some of the amazing capabilities of other visual structures. People with damage to the visual cortex cannot recognize a face or identify an apple held in front of them. However, if you put them in a room full of furniture and tell them to come to you, they will walk through the room without bumping into a single object. Place them before a computer screen with objects moving in different directions and they will say they see nothing. But ask them to follow an object with their finger and they will do it without awareness that they are successful. This phenomenon is called blind sight. Blind sight is the ability to see objects without conscious awareness of the object. Studies on people with blind sight reveal that the occipital cortex is necessary for conscious awareness of what is seen, but other structures code where the object is. Tracking a moving object occurs without conscious awareness. Neurons in the midbrain, and the superior colliculus in particular, are necessary for blind sight to occur.

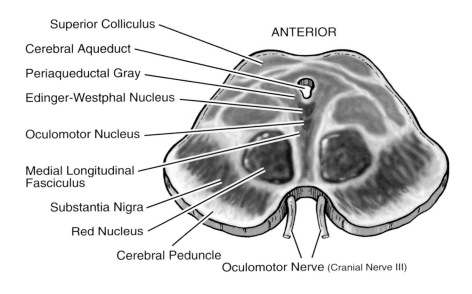

Superior Colliculus

Cerebral Aqueduct

Periaqueductal Gray

Edinger-Westphal Nucleus

Oculomotor Nucleus

Medial Longitudinal
Fasciculus

Substantia Nigra

Red Nucleus

Cerebral Peduncle

ANTERIOR

Oculomotor Nerve (Cranial Nerve III)

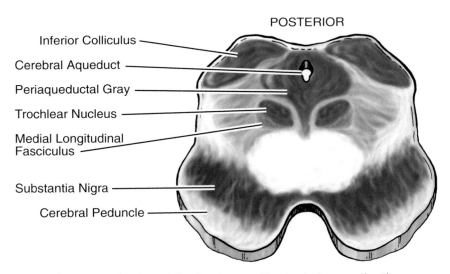

POSTERIOR

Inferior Colliculus

Cerebral Aqueduct

Periaqueductal Gray

Trochlear Nucleus

Medial Longitudinal
Fasciculus

Substantia Nigra

Cerebral Peduncle

Figure 5.1 Structures in the midbrain play a critical role in coordinating eye movements. The superior colliculus and oculomotor nucleus, including cranial nerve III descending from the oculomotor nucleus, are evident in the anterior midbrain. The Edinger-Westphal nucleus is part of the oculomotor nucleus, but controls the size of the pupil and shape of the lens. The posterior midbrain contains the trochlear nucleus and the medial longitudinal fasciculus that connects the various structures involved in eye movements.

SUPERIOR COLLICULUS

The superior colliculus appears as two large mounds protruding from the top of the midbrain. The inferior colliculus (Chapter 4) is located immediately behind, and the periaqueductal gray (Chapter 6) is located below, the superior colliculus. **Ganglion cells** in the retina of the eye simultaneously process visual images through a thalamic/cortical pathway and a midbrain pathway involving the pretectal area and superior colliculus (Figure 5.2). The superior colliculus also receives input from the auditory and somatosensory systems (**somatosensation** is the sense of touch in the skin). Auditory and somatosensory information is used to alert you to objects of interest. The superior colliculus directs your eyes to these objects. Neurons in the superior colliculus also are sensitive to visual stimuli that move. Peripheral vision is particularly good at identifying objects that move—a useful system in a world full of predators approaching from behind. Detection of these objects is easy to demonstrate. Move a feather back and forth to the side of a cat's head. Even when the object seems to be beyond the range of the eyes, the cat will know the object is there and turn its head to look at it. Thus, regardless of the stimulus—auditory, somatosensory, or visual—the superior colliculus directs the eyes to attend to it.

Of course, the superior colliculus does far more than merely direct the eyes to objects of interest. The superior colliculus also coordinates eye movements with movements of the head. The superior colliculus accomplishes this by sending messages to structures controlling the muscles that move the eyes and head. Eye movements are controlled by an output to the interstitial nucleus of Cajal (discussed later in this chapter) that projects to structures that control eye muscles (e.g., oculomotor, trochlear, and **abducens** nuclei). Head movements are coordinated by an output to reticular nuclei that control neurons in the medulla

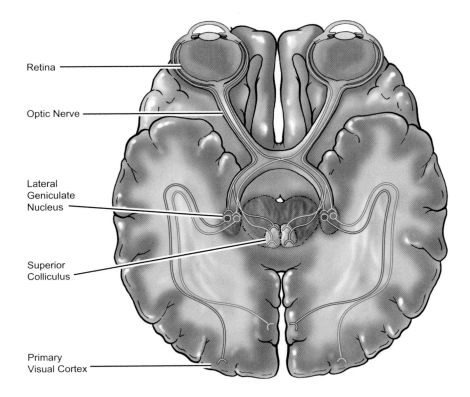

Retina

Optic Nerve

Lateral
Geniculate
Nucleus

Superior
Colliculus

Primary
Visual Cortex

Figure 5.2 Light entering the eye has several effects mediated by different pathways. Perception of the image is mediated by a pathway running from the retina to the lateral geniculate nucleus in the thalamus that relays the message to the primary visual cortex in the occipital lobe. A second pathway projects from the retina to the pretectal area and superior colliculus in the midbrain. This pathway coordinates eye and head movements so objects can be followed as they or you move. Movement of the eye is mediated by two other midbrain structures, the oculomotor and trochlear nuclei.

and spinal cord that produce head movements. Reciprocal connections to other structures involved in movement such as the basal ganglia, cerebellum, and substantia nigra (see Chapter 3) allow the superior colliculus to coordinate eye and head movements to both voluntary and involuntary movements.

PRETECTAL AREA

Given that the superior colliculus is analogous to the optic tectum in birds and fish, the term *pretectum* indicates that the pretectal area is located adjacent to and in front of the superior colliculus. Neurons in the pretectal area are grouped into discrete
clusters involved in a variety of distinct visual reflexes. These
include the pupillary reflex, the optokinetic reflex, and saccadic
eye movements. The pupillary reflex is the constriction of the
pupil that occurs when bright light enters the eye. Light activates cells in the retina that project to pretectal area neurons,
which in turn activate the Edinger-Westphal nucleus on both
sides of the brain. The Edinger-Westphal nucleus causes the
pupil to contract to limit the amount of light entering the eye
(see "Pupillary Light Reflex" box).

A different set of neurons in the pretectal area mediate the
optokinetic reflex. Optokinetic means "visual movement." A
slow-moving object casts an image on different parts of the retina as the object moves. The pretectal nucleus stabilizes this
image and sends output messages to motor pathways (vestibu-
locerebellar pathway) involved in head movements. This reflex
allows you to track the object. The eye tracks fast-moving
objects by a different mechanism. The focal point of the eye
jumps from one spot to the next by making rapid eye movements. These rapid eye movements are called saccades and
occur automatically so you can keep the moving object in focus.
Neurons in the pretectal area are connected to brain structures
involved in eye movements and to the lateral geniculate nucleus. The lateral geniculate nucleus is the target of retinal neurons
before the image is transferred to the visual cortex. Input from
the pretectal area allows synchronization of eye movements and
image so the object appears to move continuously as opposed to
jumping from spot to spot.

■ **Learn more about eye movements** Search the Internet for
superior colliculus, *saccadic*, and *vision vestibular*.

CRANIAL NERVES

Twelve pairs of **cranial nerves** provide all of the information that enters and leaves the head. This information includes sensory systems such as smell, taste, and vision, and motor systems that control the muscles that turn the head, move the tongue, and create facial expressions. The complexity of the visual system is evident in that six of the twelve cranial nerves contribute to vision (Table 5.1). Visual information enters the brain through the optic nerve (cranial nerve II) that projects directly to the superior colliculus and the lateral geniculate nucleus in the thalamus. The lateral geniculate nucleus projects to the visual cortex, which processes visual images and allows for the conscious

Pupillary Light Reflex

The pupillary light reflex is easy to observe. Stand with your face approximately six inches from a mirror in a dimly lit room. Turn on the light and watch your pupils change from large dark holes to small spots. This reflex is caused by light entering the eye. Ganglion cells in the retina respond to light by sending a message to the pretectal area in the midbrain. The pretectal area relays the message to the Edinger-Westphal nucleus on both the right and left sides of the brain. The Edinger-Westphal nucleus sends a message to the *ciliary ganglion*, which causes the iris to contract, enlarging the pupil. Because the message is sent to the Edinger-Westphal nucleus on both the right and left sides of the brain, this reflex occurs in both eyes even when light only enters one eye. You can try this experiment by looking at your left eye in a mirror in a dimly lit room. Shine a flashlight into your right eye and watch the pupil in your left eye constrict. A physician will do this experiment as part of a normal physical exam to determine whether the neurons in your retina and midbrain are functioning properly.

Table 5.1. Cranial Nerves

Number	Name	Function
I	Olfactory	Olfactory input (smell) from the nose
II	*Optic	Visual input from the eyes
III	*Oculomotor	Movement of the eyes
IV	*Trochlear	Downward movement of the eyes
V	Trigeminal	Somatosensation (touch) from the face; also muscles for chewing
VI	*Abducens	Lateral movement of the eyes
VII	Facial	Controls facial muscles and contributes to taste
VIII	Vestibulocochlear	Balance and audition (hearing) from the ear
IX	Glossopharyngeal	Controls throat muscles and contributes to taste
X	Vagus	Input and output to internal organs; sensory from viscera
XI	*Spinal accessory	Controls head and neck muscles
XII	*Hypoglossal	Controls tongue and neck muscles

* Denotes nerves that contribute to the visual system.

awareness of objects. The other five cranial nerves involved in vision control muscles that move the eyes and head. Two of these nerves, the oculomotor and trochlear, originate from nuclei located in the midbrain.

The midbrain also receives indirect input from the three other cranial nerves involved in vision—the abducens, spinal accessory, and hypoglossal nerves. The spinal accessory and hypoglossal nerves control neck muscles that allow for the synchronization of eye and head movements. In the absence of such coordination, the entire world would appear to bounce with every step taken or any movement of the head. Instead, a stable image of the world is maintained regardless of how you move. The superior colliculus is a key structure in coordinating the cranial nerves that control eye and head movements. The fiber system connecting the superior colliculus to these motor nuclei is called the **medial longitudinal fasciculus** (Chapter 8).

■ **Learn more about cranial nerves** Search the Internet for *cranial nerves* or the name of a specific nerve (see Table 5.1).

OCULOMOTOR AND TROCHLEAR NUCLEI

The superior colliculus coordinates eye movements by directly regulating the activity of three cranial nerves: the oculomotor, trochlear, and abducens. The oculomotor and trochlear nuclei are small structures embedded into the bottom of the periaqueductal gray in the midbrain. The oculomotor nucleus is especially important because it controls four of the six muscles that move the eye. The two other muscles, the superior oblique and lateral rectus, are controlled by the trochlear and abducens nuclei, respectively (Figure 5.3). These muscles allow the eyes to move right and left and up and down. Damage to the oculomotor nerve makes it impossible to follow a moving object or to move your eyes smoothly from object to object (or word to word if you are trying to read). Damage to the trochlear nerve is less severe, but results in an inability to direct your eyes downward. Patients with such damage have a very difficult time walking down stairs.

The oculomotor and trochlear nuclei are involved in a wide range of eye movements. These eye movements are involuntary and occur without conscious awareness. Even a simple task such as holding your gaze on an object requires adjusting the eyes with movements of the head. The eye muscles controlled by the oculomotor nucleus also contribute to more complicated eye movements such as smooth pursuit and vergence. Smooth pursuit is the ability to follow a slow-moving object. Fast-moving objects are tracked by rapid eye movements called saccades, as previously mentioned. Vergence is the ability to

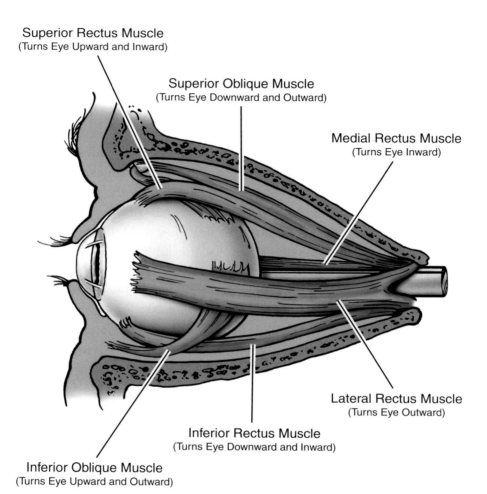

Superior Rectus Muscle
(Turns Eye Upward and Inward)

Superior Oblique Muscle
(Turns Eye Downward and Outward)

Medial Rectus Muscle
(Turns Eye Inward)

Lateral Rectus Muscle
(Turns Eye Outward)

Inferior Rectus Muscle
(Turns Eye Downward and Inward)

Inferior Oblique Muscle
(Turns Eye Upward and Outward)

Figure 5.3 The various movements of the eye require many muscles to pull the eyeball in one direction or another. The oculomotor nucleus in the midbrain controls most of these muscles (i.e., superior rectus, medial rectus, inferior rectus, and inferior oblique). Another midbrain structure, the trochlear nucleus, controls the superior oblique. This muscle pulls the eyeball down. Damage to the trochlear nucleus or superior oblique results in difficulty looking down. The only remaining muscle is the lateral rectus. This muscle is controlled by the abducens nucleus located in the pons.

focus both eyes on an object whether it is close or far. An extreme inward rotation of both eyes is required to see an object close to your nose compared to a distant object for which both eyes are directed nearly straight ahead. This coordination of the two eyes is mediated by the oculomotor nucleus. Damage to the oculomotor nucleus or a weak eye muscle will cause double vision (diplopia) because the two eyes will focus on different objects.

The Edinger-Westphal nucleus is a small subsection of the oculomotor nucleus. The function of the Edinger-Westphal nucleus is distinct from the eye movements mediated by the oculomotor nucleus in that it controls the size of the pupil and the shape of the lens. The pupil is the hole that allows light into the eye. The size of the pupil is small in bright light, but becomes large when it is dark to allow more light in (see "Pupillary Light Reflex" box). The size of the pupil is determined by the size of a small muscle called the iris. Pigment in the iris is what makes brown eyes brown and blue eyes blue. The size of this muscle is controlled by neurons in the **ciliary ganglion** that in turn is controlled by the Edinger-Westphal nucleus (Figure 5.4). The Edinger-Westphal nucleus also controls the shape of the lens. The lens is located directly behind the pupil and focuses light onto the retina. If the lens does not focus light appropriately, then artificial lenses (e.g., glasses, contact lenses) can be used to improve vision.

INTERSTITIAL NUCLEUS OF CAJAL

The interstitial nucleus of Cajal is another midbrain structure that contributes to eye movements. In particular, this structure triggers compensatory eye movements in response to head movements. The vestibular nuclei send signals about the velocity of head movements to the interstitial nucleus of Cajal. This information is integrated with input about eye movements. The

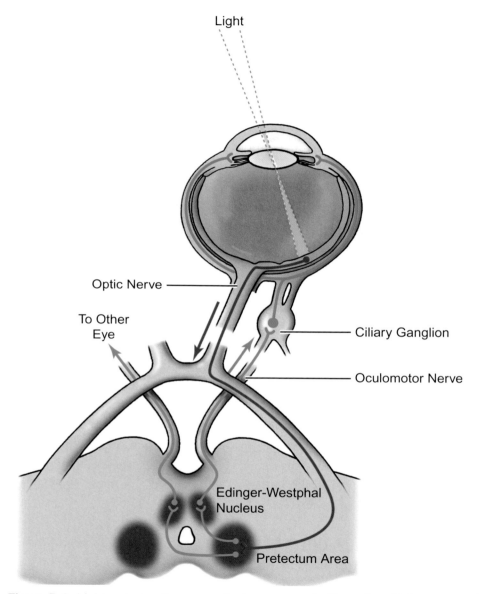

Figure 5.4 Light entering the eye activates neurons in the retina. This message is sent along the optic nerve to the pretectal area on the same side of the brain as the eye that was stimulated. The pretectal area sends the message to the Edinger-Westphal nucleus on both sides of the midbrain. The Edinger-Westphal nucleus activates the ciliary ganglion that causes the pupil to contract in both eyes. This reflex regulates how much light enters the eye. The pupil is large at night so more light enters the eye and you can see better.

interstitial nucleus of Cajal relays compensatory signals to structures such as the oculomotor and trochlear nuclei so eye movements match head movements.

SUMMARY

All of the midbrain structures involved in vision, from the superior colliculus and interstitial nucleus of Cajal to the oculomotor and trochlear nuclei, contribute to the extraordinarily complex task of producing eye movements that allow moving objects to be followed. This system also allows vision to be stable despite constant movement of the head. These movements occur quickly and without conscious thought or awareness. Although recognition of objects requires processing by the cerebral cortex, the visual system would be useless without the control of eye movements provided by the midbrain. A visual system lacking the midbrain is like giving a monkey a camera. The monkey will take pictures, but it will not make sense of the images.

6 Defense: The Real Story of *Survivor*

Joy and anxiety are the most common emotions associated with family reunions. Thus, I was surprised when fear became one of my emotions at my wife's family reunion. In addition to being nervous about meeting all of my wife's relatives, I was uneasy because one of her cousins had had her wallet stolen from her hotel room earlier in the day. I went to bed with these concerns in my mind. Around 2:00 A.M., I was awakened by a sound from across the room. I glanced toward the sound and saw a pair of legs extending down from the window (the upper body was covered by the curtains). Instantly, I jumped to my feet and stood completely naked in a fight position—legs bent, arms extended—in the middle of the bed and yelled, "Hey! Hey! Hey!" My intent was to scare the person away, but I was ready to fight if necessary. Instead of going out the window, the person turned, pulled the curtains away, and began laughing hysterically. I was shocked, and simultaneously relieved, to see that the person I thought was breaking into the room was my wife. She had woken up because she was hot and had gone to the window to turn on the air conditioning. Because it was dark in the room, she pulled the curtains over her body so she could adjust the air conditioner using the outside light. Waking someone up in the middle of the night is usually a long and difficult chore.

However, in this situation I was completely alert and ready to fight in seconds. My heart was pounding, my eyes were wide open, my body assumed a defensive position, and I yelled. These are natural defensive reactions coordinated by a midbrain structure called the periaqueductal gray matter.

This chapter is about the role of the periaqueductal gray in defensive behaviors. Unlike the television show *Survivor*, where surviving means not getting voted off the show, the periaqueductal gray allows you to survive real dangers.

PERIAQUEDUCTAL GRAY SUBDIVISIONS

The name "periaqueductal gray" is a mouthful. However, when broken into its parts the name is actually quite simple. "Peri" is Latin for "around" or "to encircle" (e.g., perimeter, periphery). "Aqueductal" refers to the cerebral aqueduct that carries cerebrospinal fluid through the midbrain. "Gray" refers to the color of a collection of cell bodies (in contrast, a collection of axons has a white appearance). Thus, the periaqueductal gray, or PAG, is a group of cell bodies that surrounds the cerebral aqueduct. The PAG runs the entire length of the midbrain and is easily visualized as a dark area surrounding the entire length of the aqueduct.

A surprising discovery was that the PAG could be divided into several different structures with different functions. These subdivisions are defined by their location. The ventrolateral subdivision is located along the lateral edges at the bottom, or ventral, part of the PAG. The lateral subdivision is located on each side of the aqueduct just above the ventrolateral region. The dorsal (top) subdivision is located directly above the aqueduct, and the dorsolateral subdivision is located between the lateral and dorsal regions (see Figure 6.1). Each of these subdivisions appears as a column that runs from front to back immediately adjacent to the aqueduct. This chapter will focus on the lateral and ven-

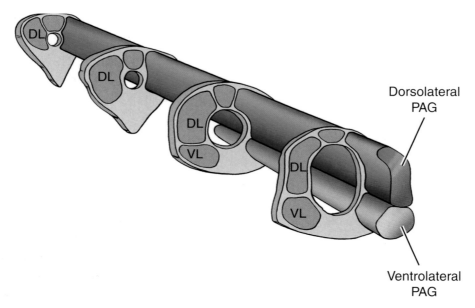

Dorsolateral
PAG

Ventrolateral
PAG

Figure 6.1 The PAG of the rat can be divided into functionally distinct columns that run the entire length of the midbrain. The lateral PAG column mediates defensive fight or flight responses, whereas the ventrolateral PAG mediates defensive immobility. Analgesia accompanies either behavioral response. The aversive reactions produced by activation of the human PAG suggest a similar organization.

trolateral subdivisions because these areas are known to contribute to defensive behaviors.

DEFENSE

The defensive reaction described at the beginning of this chapter is a classic example of what is called a fight or flight response. My entire body was on alert and ready to fight an intruder. However, if I had been outside and a swarm of bees had attacked, the defensive reaction known as flight would have occurred. The physiological response is the same for both fight and flight. Heart rate and respiration increase, blood is routed from the stomach and internal organs to the muscles, the pupils dilate to enhance peripheral vision, and the hair on the back of your neck stands up (this is called piloerection and is very

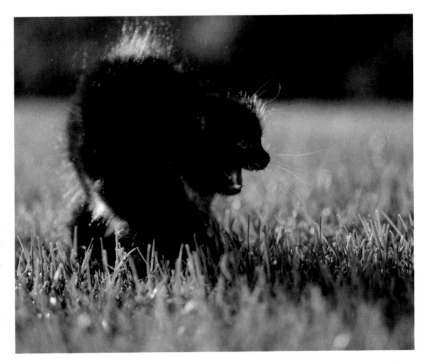

Figure 6.2 Everyone recognizes the emotions displayed by the cat often depicted at Halloween: arched back, raised hair, lowered ears, and hissing are clear signs that the cat is frightened. This defensive response is organized by the periaqueductal gray in the midbrain. Although differences in defense exist between animals, cardiovascular and other changes are common. In fact, check the hair on the back of your neck the next time you are frightened—it will probably be standing up.

noticeable when cats and dogs are frightened (Figure 6.2). In addition, pain sensitivity decreases, a response known as **analgesia**. These responses allow animals to do whatever is necessary to survive. An increase in heart rate, respiration, and dilation of blood vessels in the muscles allows more oxygen to reach the muscles to facilitate running and fighting. Analgesia facilitates escape and survival by preventing injuries from distracting the animal. Thus, the physiological changes associated with the fight or flight response provide both the energy and analgesia necessary to survive. Intense athletic competition can produce the same physiological changes, including analgesia. However, once the threat (or game) has passed, the pain from any cuts and bruises will be felt.

FIGHT OR FLIGHT AND THE LATERAL PAG

Fight or flight is a complicated behavior that involves many brain structures. The lateral PAG receives input from structures such as the amygdala, hypothalamus, and spinal cord, and then organizes the various components of the defensive response. Direct electrical or chemical activation of neurons in the lateral PAG of the rat produces the same physiological response as naturally occurring threats. There is an increase in heart rate and respiration and a shift in blood flow from internal organs to muscles. These physiological changes are accompanied by distress vocalizations, analgesia, and explosive running and jumping. The running response is so profound that it is almost impossible to catch these rats if they get out of their cage. Stimulation of the PAG in humans produces similar effects and is reported to be quite unpleasant (see "PAG Stimulation in Humans" box).

Studies examining natural stimuli that produce escape responses also point to the lateral PAG as a key structure in mediating this response. Escape responses can be evoked by injury to the neck, and application of such stimuli activates neurons in the lateral PAG. In addition, inactivation of the lateral PAG prevents the fight or flight response.

FREEZING AND THE VENTROLATERAL PAG

Of course, defensive reactions are effective only if they vary with the specific situation. The cerebral cortex evaluates the situation and sends a message regarding the magnitude of the threat to the PAG. If hiding behind a tree is sufficient to ensure survival,

PAG Stimulation in Humans

Imagine the worst pain you have ever experienced (e.g., a broken bone or burn). Some chronic pain patients live for years with pain sensations this intense. Although some of these patients can be treated with opiates, others get no relief. In the 1970s, neurosurgeons tried a radical treatment to help these people—intracranial brain stimulation. Because it was known that electrical stimulation of the PAG in rats produced analgesia, the assumption was that such stimulation might work in people. The surgery consisted of lowering an electrode into the brain while the patient was awake so the most effective site in blocking pain could be located (there are no pain receptors in the brain, so a local anesthetic on the skin and bone is all that was necessary). Once an effective site was identified, the electrode was fixed to the skull and a connecting wire was run under the skin to a control box attached to the chest. Patients managed their pain by pushing a button on the control box to activate the PAG. Although PAG stimulation reduced pain, it also produced unpleasant sensations. These sensations appeared to come from within the body (e.g., chest, throat, bladder) and were accompanied by fear, anxiety, and a sense of danger. One patient described the feeling as "fearful, frightful, and terrible," and he would not allow further stimulations. In another patient, PAG stimulation caused a feeling that "Something horrible is coming. Somebody is now chasing me. I am trying to escape." These statements support the view that the analgesia produced from the PAG is part of a defense reaction, and simultaneously point out why this treatment is rarely used today.

then there is no need to engage in a fight. Rats follow the same logic even though the response is automatically controlled by the PAG. Flight normally occurs when a cat pounces on a rat. However, if the rat detects the cat prior to the pounce, the rat will become immobile. This response, also known as freezing, is a defensive strategy that aims to avoid the attack (as you know, cats and other predators prefer prey and toys that move). Analgesia accompanies both fight and flight and freezing defensive reactions. Pain is blocked during the fight or flight response so escape is possible. Analgesia accompanies freezing to prevent the muscle and joint pain that occurs with prolonged immobility. Although you rarely notice these pains because you constantly shift your body, if you stand or sit for a prolonged time you will experience pain in your muscles and joints (this pain is particularly noticeable when sitting through a long, boring lecture).

Activation of neurons in the ventrolateral PAG causes immobility. Although immobility can be associated with recuperation from injury, a lack of motivation, or a movement impairment, a number of findings suggests that the immobility mediated by the ventrolateral PAG is a defensive reaction. First, activation of the ventrolateral PAG produces analgesia, a response that is not part of recuperation. Second, inactivation of the ventrolateral PAG prevents the freezing response and analgesia produced by a naturally frightening stimulus.

Fear is the natural trigger for the freezing response. A forebrain structure called the amygdala plays an important role in emotions such as fear. The fear message generated in the amygdala is transmitted directly to the PAG, where immobility and analgesia are produced. More information about the amygdala is available in other books in this series.

■ **Learn more about defensive behaviors** Search the Internet for *defense behavior, affective defense, defensive freezing,* and *fear conditioning.*

OPIOID ANALGESIA

As mentioned previously, analgesia is an important part of defensive behavior. Analgesia is mediated by specialized neurotransmitters called **opioids**. Opioids and the receptors for opioids are located throughout the PAG. A number of natural and synthetic chemicals mimic the actions of the opioid neurotransmitters. These drugs are classified as opiates or narcotics and have names like morphine, fentanyl, and codeine. Opiates are the most powerful pain medications available.

Most of the opiates used to treat pain have a chemical structure similar to that of morphine. Morphine is a naturally occurring chemical found in opium (derived from a flower called the poppy). Once morphine enters the bloodstream, it travels throughout the circulatory system and eventually comes in contact with opioid receptors wherever they exist. A receptor is a specialized protein on the surface of a cell. Neurotransmitters bind to receptors in the same way that a key fits into a lock. Given that there are many different neurotransmitters, there are many different receptors. Thus, the different naturally occurring opioid neurotransmitters bind preferentially to different opioid receptors (see Table 6.1). Pharmaceutical companies can make drugs that bind to these receptors and produce analgesia much as a locksmith can pick the lock on the door of your house.

Analgesia occurs when morphine binds to opioid receptors in the PAG and a few other structures (e.g., **rostral ventromedial**

Table 6.1. Naturally Occurring Opioids

Opioid	Receptor	Cell Location	Analgesic Potency
Beta-endorphin	mu	Hypothalamus, Solitary tract nucleus	Strong analgesic
Enkephalin	delta	PAG, RVM, Spinal cord	Moderate analgesic
Dynorphin	kappa	PAG, RVM, Spinal cord	Weak analgesic

medulla [RVM] and spinal cord). Morphine activates neurons in the PAG that then activate neurons in the RVM. The RVM, in turn, transmits the message to the spinal cord where pain messages entering from the body are inhibited (Figure 6.3). Opiates like morphine are especially good at blocking pain because they act at all three levels of this system—the PAG, RVM, and spinal cord.

Although morphine and other opioids are great at blocking pain, their usefulness is limited because of side effects. These side effects can range from irritating (e.g., constipation) to life-threatening (e.g., respiratory depression). The side effects are caused by opiate binding to receptors located in a variety of different structures. For example, constipation is caused by opiate binding to receptors in the intestines, whereas respiratory depression is caused by opioid binding to receptors in a structure called the subretrofacial nucleus.

Morphine and other opiates are particularly dangerous because they are addictive. Opiates bind to receptors in the reward pathway to produce euphoria (see Chapter 7). Repeated administration of opiates leads to addiction because neurons try to adjust to the large amount of opiate in the body. These adjustments could be a reduction in the number of opioid receptors or a change in the intracellular molecules activated by the receptor. The net effect is a neuron that is less responsive to the drug. A decrease in effect of a drug with repeated administration is called tolerance. The need to increase the dose of morphine to reduce pain is an example of tolerance. Neurons in the ventrolateral PAG play a critical role in tolerance to the pain inhibition produced by morphine.

The adjustments made by the nervous system that cause tolerance also lead to withdrawal symptoms when the opiate is removed. Withdrawal symptoms are in the opposite direction to the effect of opiates. Thus, instead of constipation and analgesia, diarrhea and hyperalgesia (increased pain) occur.

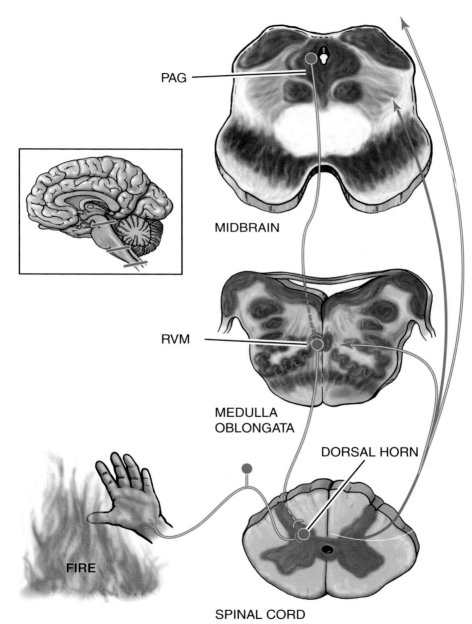

PAG

MIDBRAIN

RVM

MEDULLA
OBLONGATA

DORSAL HORN

FIRE

SPINAL CORD

Figure 6.3 The periaqueductal gray (PAG) is part of a natural system involved in modulating pain. Neurons in the PAG project to the rostral ventromedial medulla (RVM) that in turn projects to the spinal cord. Activation of this descending system inhibits pain messages as they enter the spinal cord. The RVM and spinal cord also send messages back to the PAG as part of a feedback system.

Withdrawal symptoms are often so severe that instead of removing opioids altogether, addicts are often switched from a dangerous opiate like heroin to a less dangerous opiate like methadone. Methadone prevents withdrawal symptoms by binding to opioid receptors, but does not enter the nervous system as quickly and so is less addictive and less dangerous (see "Morphine vs. Aspirin" box).

■ **Learn more about drugs that inhibit pain** Search the Internet for *opioid*, *analgesics*, *NSAIDs*, or use the name of a specific drug (e.g., fentanyl).

Morphine vs. Aspirin

Morphine and aspirin belong to a broad class of drugs called analgesics. Although both drugs reduce pain, they do so in very different ways. Opiates like morphine activate brain regions such as the PAG and RVM that inhibit pain. In addition, opiates directly inhibit pain-processing neurons in the peripheral nervous system and spinal cord. In contrast, aspirin and other non-steroidal anti-inflammatory drugs (NSAIDs) do not block pain directly, but inhibit inflammation and sensitization in neurons. NSAIDs are very effective in blocking mild aches and pains, but will not block the pain produced by surgery. Opiates are much more effective in blocking severe pain. Unfortunately, side effects limit the use of opiates. In particular, the euphoria and potential for addiction make opiates much more dangerous than NSAIDs. Thus, another difference between morphine and aspirin is that a prescription is necessary to use opiates, whereas aspirin and other NSAIDs (ibuprofen, acetaminophen) can be bought at a drug store.

INPUTS AND OUTPUTS

As mentioned previously, fear messages are transmitted to the PAG from a structure in the forebrain called the amygdala. The PAG also receives input from the cerebral cortex, hypothalamus, medulla oblongata, spinal cord, and other midbrain structures. The emotional state of the animal is relayed to the PAG from the medial **prefrontal cortex**, insular cortex, and cingulate gyrus. Information about the state of the animal's body is coordinated through the autonomic nervous system. (The autonomic nervous system is regulated by the hypothalamus and controls automatic changes in the body like heart rate, respiration, and sweating). The hypothalamus provides a massive input to the PAG. One of the neurotransmitters in the pathway from the hypothalamus to PAG is a naturally occurring opioid called beta-endorphin. Beta-endorphin, like injectable opiates, activates the PAG to produce analgesia. Visual and auditory information reach the PAG from the superior and inferior colliculi, two structures immediately above the PAG (see Chapters 4 and 5). These inputs provide the emotional, motivational, and sensory information necessary for the coordinated defensive reactions produced by the PAG. The location of these neural structures is shown in Figure 6.4.

The different aspects of the defensive reactions mediated by the PAG appear to be controlled by PAG outputs to specific targets. These include projections to the RVM for analgesia, and other medullary nuclei for cardiovascular changes and vocalization. Direct projections to deep parts of the spinal cord allow for defensive postures. Other output projections from the PAG appear to contribute to such diverse behaviors as urination (Barrington's nucleus) and mating (nucleus retroambiguus).

In most cases, the PAG receives input from the same structures to which it projects. These reciprocal connections allow feedback so behavioral responses can be adjusted as needed. For

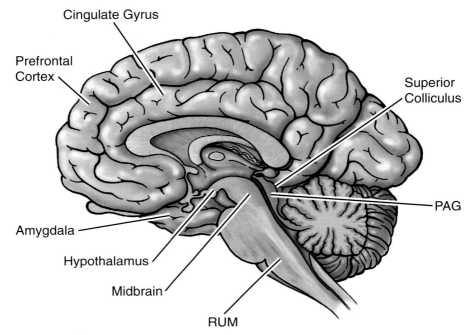

Figure 6.4 The defensive behaviors organized by the PAG are determined by inputs from many parts of the nervous system. Many of these structures can be seen on a midsagittal section of brain. Forebrain inputs include the prefrontal cortex, cingulate cortex, amygdala, and hypothalamus. The PAG also receives input from the rostral ventromedial medulla, the spinal cord, and other structures in the midbrain such as the superior and inferior colliculi.

example, the PAG modulates pain by an output to the RVM. The RVM relays this message to the spinal cord to inhibit pain. Neurons in both the RVM and spinal cord project back to the PAG so pain sensitivity can be adjusted as needed.

SUMMARY

Anatomical, pharmacological, and behavioral data indicate that the PAG plays an important role in coordinating defensive behaviors. The cardiovascular and movement changes evoked by threatening stimuli occur automatically and range from fight or flight to immobility. These responses are mediated by the lateral and ventrolateral PAG. Analgesia is an important component of these defensive reactions. Therapeutically, this system is important because opiates such as morphine produce analgesia by activating neurons in the PAG. Thus, whether you take opiates for surgery or are fighting off a bear, the PAG is an important structure.

7 Reward: Sex, Drugs, and Rock 'n' Roll

W hat do sex, drugs, and rock-n-roll have in common? Although all three are signs of teenage rebellion, the strand that links these activities is found in the brain. Sex, drugs, and good music activate regions of the brain involved in reward. The two key structures in this reward circuit are the ventral tegmental area in the midbrain and the nucleus accumbens in the forebrain. The sensation of pleasure is made possible by these two structures. Animals cannot survive without this reward circuit, and yet the behaviors people engage in to stimulate this reward circuit can be very destructive. For example, if sex were not pleasurable, it is unlikely anyone would go through the time and effort to engage in this activity. The risks associated with sex (e.g., unwanted pregnancy, sexually transmitted diseases) provide strong arguments to limit sexual behavior. Although everyone must weigh the pros and cons of engaging in sex, teenagers are at a disadvantage in making this judgment because the area of the brain involved in decision making (i.e., the frontal cortex) is not fully developed. Given that the reward circuit is developed, teenagers tend to make decisions based on pleasure without regard to the consequences. This type of brain development has not always been a problem. The relatively short life span of humans living 10,000 years ago made sex early in life a necessity for survival of the species. The surprisingly high rates of teenage pregnancy and sexually transmitted diseases in society today make this brain arrangement less than ideal. This chapter describes how the midbrain contributes to reward and examines the positive and negative consequences of this reward pathway.

VENTRAL TEGMENTAL AREA

The ventral tegmental area (VTA) is a small structure located in the lower half of the midbrain. It is immediately adjacent to the substantia nigra and is similar to the substantia nigra in that neurons in both structures contain the neurotransmitter dopamine. In fact, the substantia nigra and the VTA are the two primary sources of dopamine in the brain (Figure 7.1). Both the substantia nigra and VTA communicate with a group of structures in the forebrain known as the basal ganglia. As described in Chapter 3, the substantia nigra is involved in initiating voluntary movements through the release of dopamine in a part of the basal ganglion called the striatum. The VTA releases dopamine in a nearby part of the basal ganglia called the nucleus accumbens. This pathway mediates reward.

Psychologists define reward as anything that increases the likelihood of a behavior. This broad definition encompasses a wide range of stimuli. Rewards that are common to all animals include food and safety. Rewards more specific to humans include doing well on an exam, receiving a compliment, helping others, and falling in love. All of these things activate neurons in the VTA. The VTA relays the message to the nucleus accumbens, which creates the sensation of pleasure. The axons running from the VTA to the nucleus accumbens are part of the **mesolimbic pathway** (Figure 7.2). This pathway also includes projections to the prefrontal cortex and other forebrain structures. The mesolimbic pathway allows the brain to distinguish things that

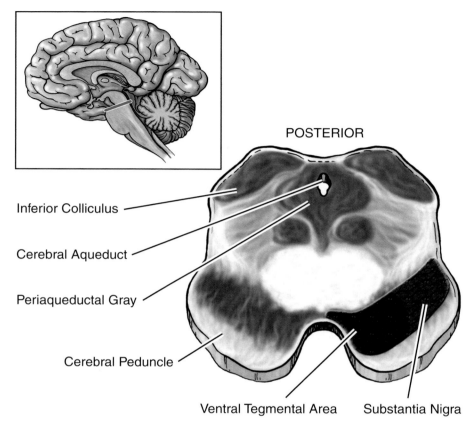

POSTERIOR

Inferior Colliculus

Cerebral Aqueduct

Periaqueductal Gray

Cerebral Peduncle

Ventral Tegmental Area   Substantia Nigra

Figure 7.1 The ventral tegmental area is located at the bottom of the midbrain. It is continuous with the substantia nigra and, like the substantia nigra, contains the neurotransmitter dopamine. The primary difference is that the ventral tegmental area is located toward the middle of the midbrain and the substantia nigra extends to the lateral edge. These structures have different functions because the ventral tegmental area projects to the nucleus accumbens (reward) and the substantia nigra projects to the striatum (movement).

are good and should be repeated from things that are bad and should be avoided.

Another name for the band of fibers that make up the mesolimbic pathway is the **medial forebrain bundle**. Although this pathway is normally activated by natural stimuli, electrical

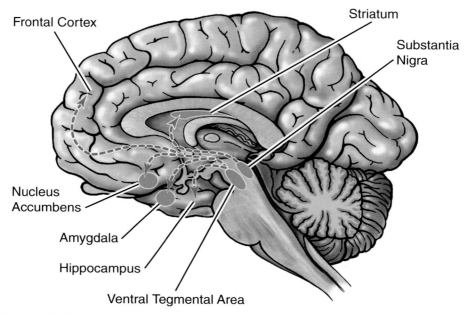

Frontal Cortex

Striatum

Substantia Nigra

Nucleus Accumbens

Amygdala

Hippocampus

Ventral Tegmental Area

Figure 7.2 The mesolimbic pathway is the reward pathway. It originates from neurons in the ventral tegmental area and projects to limbic structures such as the nucleus accumbens, hippocampus, amygdala, and frontal cortex. In contrast, the adjacent substantia nigra projects via the nigrostriatal pathway to the striatum.

stimulation of this bundle of axons is rewarding (see "Discovery of the Reward Pathway" box). The power of this reward pathway is best demonstrated by studies showing that rats prefer electrical stimulation of this circuit to any naturally occurring reward (e.g., food, sleep). In addition to rats, electrical stimulation of the medial forebrain bundle has been shown to be rewarding in cats, monkeys, and humans. In contrast, stimulation of other brain structures such as the periaqueductal gray is aversive—animals actively avoid such stimulation (see Chapter 6). Although electrical stimulation is not a natural stimulus, electrical stimulation has been very useful in identifying brain structures that signal pleasure and aversion.

Natural stimuli, whether rewarding or aversive, are transmitted to the brain by sensory systems such as vision, touch, and taste. Depending on the characteristics of the stimulus (e.g., sweet chocolate vs. sour milk), the message may or may not activate neurons in the VTA. The screening process that determines what stimuli activate the VTA is complex and poorly understood. Some stimuli are inherently rewarding (e.g., milk and touch in babies), whereas other rewards are learned (e.g., money). Regardless of whether the stimulus is a natural or learned reward, activation of VTA neurons causes the release of dopamine onto neurons in the nucleus accumbens. The release of dopamine in the nucleus accumbens is a key step in signaling reward.

Discovery of the Reward Pathway

In the early 1950s, James Olds and a graduate student, Peter Milner, began electrically stimulating the rat brain in the hope of identifying structures that would facilitate learning. They aimed their stimulating electrode at the reticular formation in the back of the brain and missed badly. Instead of stimulating the reticular formation, they stimulated the medial forebrain bundle, a collection of axons running from the VTA to the forebrain. Unlike rats receiving stimulation of the reticular formation, rats receiving stimulation of the medial forebrain bundle eagerly returned to the test chamber whenever the opportunity presented itself. Thus, Olds and Milner modified the experiment so the rat could press a lever to receive electrical stimulation of the medial forebrain bundle—a phenomenon known as self-stimulation. With just a few jolts of electricity to prime the rat, the rat began to rapidly press the lever and would not stop. Through both accident and insight, Olds and Milner had discovered the reward pathway in the brain.

■ **Learn more about reward systems in the brain** Search the Internet for *brain reward, nucleus accumbens pleasure,* and *medial forebrain bundle.*

OTHER STRUCTURES CONTRIBUTING TO REWARD

Although the primary pathway for reward runs from the VTA to the nucleus accumbens, other structures contribute to reward by modifying this message. For example, food is rewarding only if you are hungry. Food is not rewarding 30 minutes after a huge Thanksgiving meal. Thus, even though the stimulus is the same, the response of neurons in the nucleus accumbens can be muted. Three forebrain structures, the amygdala, hippocampus, and prefrontal cortex, are important in modifying the reward message.

The amygdala is a small structure buried within the temporal lobe of the cerebral cortex. It codes emotions ranging from anxiety and fear to happiness. Unlike the VTA to nucleus accumbens pathway, the amygdala contributes to both pleasure and fear. Thus, the amygdala helps determine whether a stimulus should be approached or avoided and triggers physiological changes (e.g., heart rate, respiration) consistent with each emotion.

The hippocampus is adjacent to the amygdala, but it is a much longer structure, looping away from the amygdala along the inner edge of the temporal cortex. The hippocampus is involved in the creation and retrieval of memories. Past memories have a profound effect on what is rewarding. The curiosity that drives learning is normally a rewarding experience. However, if you are teased every time you go to school to learn, then the reward value of learning is diminished. The hippocampus modulates reward by providing memories of the consequences of past experience.

The **prefrontal cortex** contributes to reward by predicting the consequences of a particular behavior. This is accomplished by evaluating past experiences, the reward value of the stimulus, and current emotional and motivational states. If you are hungry and past experiences with chocolate have been positive, then the prefrontal cortex will send a signal to eat the chocolate. One of the most surprising recent findings in neuroscience is that the prefrontal cortex continues to develop throughout the teenage years. As you know from observing friends at school, teenagers make more than their share of bad decisions. These poor decisions can be blamed in part on the fact that the frontal cortex is not functioning at full capacity, and thus, may not counter the power of the reward circuit.

■ **Learn more about brain development in adolescents** Search the Internet for *adolescent prefrontal cortex.*

The VTA projects directly to the amygdala, hippocampus, and prefrontal cortex in addition to the strong direct projection to the nucleus accumbens. The amygdala, hippocampus, and prefrontal cortex also project to the nucleus accumbens. Thus, the activity of neurons in the VTA signals the magnitude of reward to all four of these structures. The amygdala, hippocampus, and prefrontal cortex modulate this message by sending a message about the current emotional state, past experience, and expected outcome of responding to the stimulus to the nucleus accumbens. In addition, neurons in the nucleus accumbens send messages back to the VTA to adjust neural activity. In this way, the magnitude of the reward associated with a particular stimulus is adjusted. This is an ideal circuit in that it integrates all the factors necessary for determining the degree of pleasure produced by a particular stimulus, including a feedback mechanism to adjust the signal.

DRUG ABUSE

The pathway from the VTA to the nucleus accumbens is particularly important in understanding why people abuse drugs. All drugs of abuse from alcohol to amphetamine to heroin mimic natural rewards by activating the mesolimbic reward circuit. Given that the VTA produces reward by releasing dopamine onto neurons in the nucleus accumbens, drugs that increase dopamine will be rewarding, and thus are likely to be abused. The amount of dopamine acting on neurons can be modified in many ways. Amphetamine triggers VTA neurons to release dopamine. Cocaine blocks removal of dopamine. Normally, dopamine is released by VTA neurons, binds to receptors on neurons in the nucleus accumbens, and then is removed by being taken back into the VTA neuron (a natural recycling program). Binding to the receptor is short-lived, so the effects of dopamine are transient. Cocaine prolongs the effect of dopamine by blocking this reuptake mechanism (Figure 7.3).

The activity of VTA neurons is kept under control by neurons containing a neurotransmitter called GABA. GABA inhibits VTA neurons so reward signals are not sent continuously. Alcohol and opiates such as heroin reduce the activity of these GABA-containing neurons. Inhibition of the GABA neuron causes the VTA neuron to become active, resulting in dopamine release in the nucleus accumbens. Thus, opiates and alcohol are rewarding and commonly abused. Other drugs, like nicotine, activate VTA neurons directly. Table 7.1 provides a list of abused drugs and the presumed neural mechanism.

The reason these drugs are abused is that they hijack the reward system. Natural stimuli activate this system in a very discrete manner, causing dopamine to be released and removed as needed. In contrast, drugs enter the bloodstream and remain in the system for hours. As long as the drug is in the blood it will

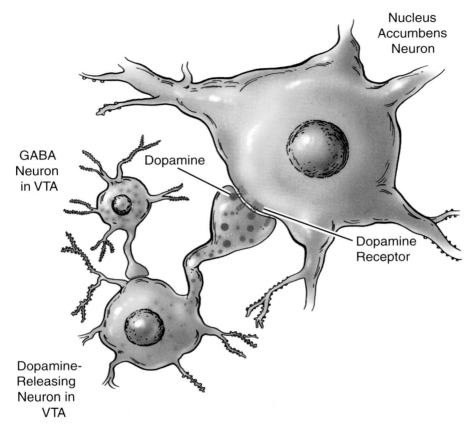

Figure 7.3 There are three types of neurons that drugs of abuse act on. Neurons in the ventral tegmental area release dopamine onto neurons in the nucleus accumbens. The activity of the ventral tegmental area neurons is controlled by GABA-containing neurons in the VTA. Drugs of abuse act on one of these three neurons to increase dopamine in the nucleus accumbens. Some drugs inhibit the GABA neuron (e.g., heroin). Other drugs activate the VTA neuron directly (nicotine). Other drugs stimulate the release of dopamine in the nucleus accumbens (amphetamine).

continue to activate VTA neurons. Thus, neurons in the nucleus accumbens are exposed to prolonged high levels of dopamine. This persistent activation produces an enhanced feeling of reward and simultaneously alters the normal functioning of the reward circuit.

Table 7.1. Drugs of Abuse

Drug	Mechanism
Amphetamine	Releases dopamine from VTA neurons
Cocaine	Blocks dopamine reuptake into VTA neurons
Heroin	Releases dopamine by inhibiting GABA neurons in VTA
Alcohol	Releases dopamine by inhibiting GABA neurons in VTA
Nicotine	Releases dopamine by stimulating VTA neurons

Note: these drugs have additional effects to the ones listed in this table.

The nervous system is a surprisingly well-tuned machine that adjusts its activity depending on prior activity. Problems occur when there is too little or too much activity. Drugs that cause high levels of dopamine in the nucleus accumbens trigger feedback mechanisms that counteract the effect of the drug. For example, high dopamine levels are offset by a reduction in dopamine synthesis in VTA neurons and a decrease in responsiveness to dopamine in nucleus accumbens neurons. When the effect of the drug ends, the activity of the mesolimbic reward circuit becomes less active than normal, which dampens the sense of reward. This feeling can lead to additional drug taking to regain the feeling of pleasure—a phenomenon known as addiction.

Chronic drug use also leads to dependence. Dependence means that the body can no longer function without the drug. That is, neurons become so accustomed to a drug that they do not function properly if the drug is not present. Without the drug, withdrawal symptoms occur. Withdrawal symptoms can be mild, like the headache that occurs with the cessation of chronic caffeine consumption, or severe, as occurs with the pain and suffering of heroin withdrawal. Heroin withdrawal is so miserable and severe that most people cannot quit. These people are switched to a much less dangerous opiate called methadone in order to function in daily life.

The problem with drug addiction is that all other stimuli that produce reward become secondary to the reward produced by the drug. People lose interest in food, friends, work, and safety. The rewards that come from these activities cannot compete with the powerful activation of the mesolimbic reward circuit produced by drugs of abuse. It is particularly interesting that rats will abuse the same drugs as humans if given the opportunity. Rats will self-administer these drugs in exclusion of food and even when it endangers their safety. In this way, humans and rats look very similar. In fact, much has been learned about drug addiction from studies using rats. One of the most frightening findings is that even after prolonged abstinence from drug taking, changes in the mesolimbic reward circuit persist. Thus, drug relapse is a serious problem that can occur years after drug use has stopped.

Studies examining brain activity in living humans show that drugs of abuse activate the nucleus accumbens. Similar activation occurs by merely presenting stimuli associated with drug use such as a needle and syringe. These effects can last for months after drug use has ended. In addition, the nucleus accumbens is activated in people addicted to gambling when shown stimuli associated with gambling (e.g., cards, slot machines). These studies indicate that the VTA-to-nucleus accumbens reward circuit contributes to all types of addictions.

■ **Learn more about drug abuse** Search the Internet for *drug abuse* and the names of specific drugs (e.g., alcohol, nicotine, and heroin).

SUMMARY

The VTA and the dopamine contained in these neurons are the central component of the reward system. Natural stimuli that cause VTA neurons to release dopamine are rewarding, which makes you likely to engage in those behaviors again. However, this reward system also can lead to behaviors like drug abuse and gambling, which are destructive. The fact that many people engage in these destructive behaviors demonstrates the power of the reward circuit.

8 Fibers: Before the Wireless Revolution

The capabilities of computers are rapidly catching up to and overtaking human abilities. Computers can recognize your voice and speak to you, vacuum your house, and defeat the best chess players in the world. These examples demonstrate that a single computer can outperform a human on a specific task, but computers are surprisingly incompetent when compared to the wide range of abilities of a human (e.g., the chess-playing computer would be destroyed if it tried to ride a bike). The wireless revolution, in which computers do not need to be connected by wires, will allow much more versatile computers. In fact, networks of computers, each programmed for a specific task, can work together in much the same way structures of the brain work together. The nervous system has specialized structures to detect stimuli (e.g., the retina detects light), produce movements (e.g., the oculomotor nucleus moves the eye), and integrate these responses (e.g., the superior colliculus coordinates eye and head movements). Specialized computers connected through a network can perform similar tasks, but will accomplish it through wireless communication. In contrast, the structures in the brain rely on wires to communicate. The "wires" in the human brain are the axons that carry messages from neuron to neuron. These axons are often bundled together into large tracts that are easily visible as they pass through the brain and body. These axon bundles are the most prominent feature in the midbrain (see "Models of the Brain" box).

Chapters 2 through 7 focused on the various nuclei located in the midbrain. These groups of neurons stand out in a coronal section because they are dark (i.e., gray matter). Thus, most of the other structures in the midbrain must be axons (i.e., white matter) (Figure 8.1). These axons are white because of the myelin sheath that wraps around to form insulation—much as electrical wires are insulated. Myelin allows electrical signals to travel rapidly and across great distances within an axon (some axons are six feet long traveling from the toe to the brain). Electrical signals would leak from the axon and stop if the myelin sheath breaks down. Multiple sclerosis is a disorder in which the myelin sheath breaks down, causing a wide range of problems such as difficulty walking, talking, and feeling stimuli.

Many of the axons in the midbrain are merely traveling through without communicating with local nuclei. (Imagine an express freeway with no off-ramps). Other axons are part of the input and output through which the structures in the midbrain communicate with other structures. These connections can be entirely within the midbrain or with structures outside the midbrain. The remainder of this chapter will describe both types of midbrain connections and provide insights about their functions.

■ **Learn more about axons** Search the Internet for *white matter, myelin sheath,* and *neuronal axon.*

JUST PASSING THROUGH

The **cerebral peduncles** are the most massive fiber bundle in the brain. These fibers pass through the midbrain on the way from the cerebral cortex to the pons, medulla, and spinal cord. The cerebral peduncles are located along the bottom of the midbrain directly below the substantia nigra and ventral tegmental area. Each peduncle is made up of approximately 20 million axons

Models of the Brain

The complexity of the brain makes it extremely difficult to understand. Models of the brain can provide a better understanding of the brain, assuming the model is accurate. René Descartes proposed a hydraulic model of the brain in the 17th century. The movement of fluids from one place to another can cause objects to move, and Descartes had dissected enough humans to know about the fluid-filled ventricles of the brain. Subsequent scientists realized that nerves were not hollow tubes and that messages were transmitted by electricity, so the hydraulic model was dropped. The development of the telephone switchboard in the 19th century provided a new model of the brain. A switchboard allows people in one house to be connected to people in another house by inserting a wire into the appropriate locations on the switchboard. The idea that structures in the brain are connected by wires is accurate, but these connections are automatically determined during development and take a long time to change, if they can change at all. The computer is the preferred model from the 20th century. A computer has a well-protected "brain" called the central processing unit (CPU) that converts input (striking a key) into output (a word on the screen). Despite these similarities, the computer is a shockingly simple model. Although the brain lacks the processing speed of a computer, it compensates by being able to do many things well and adjusting output depending on past experiences and current conditions. Perhaps the model for the 21st century will be computer networks in which each computer functions as a specific nucleus in communication with other nuclei. This type of model may be able to replicate all human abilities. Although the idea that a machine can fully replicate human abilities is controversial, time will tell whether the computers of the future will succeed.

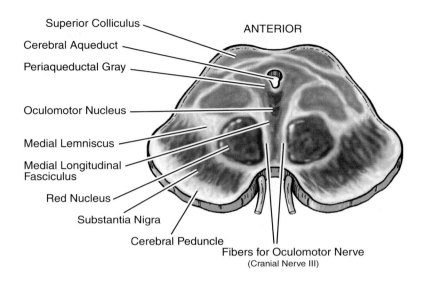

Superior Colliculus
Cerebral Aqueduct
Periaqueductal Gray

Oculomotor Nucleus

Medial Lemniscus

Medial Longitudinal
Fasciculus

Red Nucleus

Substantia Nigra

Cerebral Peduncle

ANTERIOR

Fibers for Oculomotor Nerve
(Cranial Nerve III)

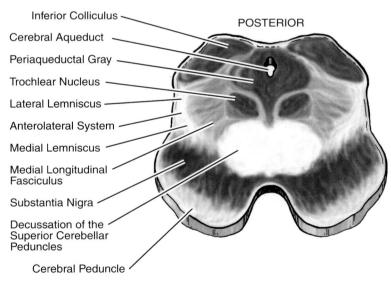

Inferior Colliculus
Cerebral Aqueduct
Periaqueductal Gray
Trochlear Nucleus
Lateral Lemniscus
Anterolateral System
Medial Lemniscus
Medial Longitudinal
Fasciculus
Substantia Nigra
Decussation of the
Superior Cerebellar
Peduncles
Cerebral Peduncle

POSTERIOR

Figure 8.1 A coronal section through the midbrain reveals several large fiber bundles. The most massive bundles of axons are the corticopontine, corticobulbar, and corticospinal tracts that make up the cerebral peduncle. Other prominent fiber bundles are the decussation of the superior cerebellar peduncles and the medial lemniscus and anterolateral pathways. Other fiber systems provide input to structures in the midbrain (e.g., lateral lemniscus), while others carry information within the midbrain (e.g., posterior commissure) or to structures outside the midbrain (e.g., oculomotor nerve).

descending from neurons in the motor cortex. The axons are named according to whether they synapse on neurons in the pons (corticopontine tract), medulla (corticobulbar tract), or spinal cord (corticospinal tract). The specific connection is to a motoneuron, a unique class of neuron that projects to a specific muscle. The corticopontine and corticobulbar tracts project to motoneurons that control muscles in the head and neck. The corticospinal tract projects to motoneurons in the spinal cord controlling the muscles in the body. Damage to different parts of the cerebral peduncle will result in a loss of voluntary movement to a specific set of muscles on the opposite side of the body from which the damage occurred.

The **medial lemniscus** and **anterolateral pathway** appear as a continuous column along the lateral edges of the midbrain. The medial lemniscus carries information about touch and joint position from the body to the brain. These fibers arise from a medullary structure called the dorsal column nuclei. The dorsal column nuclei receive input from sensory neurons originating in the skin and traveling up the spinal cord. The dorsal column nucleus on the right side of the body sends information to the thalamus on the opposite side of the brain via the medial lemniscus. Thus, anything that touches the right side of your body is coded as touch on the left side of the brain. The anterolateral pathway carries pain messages from the spinal cord to the thalamus. The axons of these spinal neurons cross to the opposite side of the spinal cord and then ascend as the anterolateral pathway (see "Neurological Exam" box).

No nuclei are located in the middle of the midbrain above and around the red nuclei. This huge space is filled by axons leaving the cerebellum, crossing to the opposite side of the body, and projecting to the thalamus. This crossing of axons is called the decussation of the **superior cerebellar peduncles**. There are three pairs of cerebellar peduncles carrying information to and from the cerebellum. The superior cerebellar peduncle from the right and left of the cerebellum cross in the midbrain. These fibers carry information to the thalamus and motor cortex to assist in the coordination and production of movement. The axons from the right and left sides are intermingled as they cross in the midbrain, leaving this region poorly defined compared to the cerebral peduncles or medial lemniscus.

Neurological Exam

Neurologists are physicians who specialize in treating disorders of the nervous system. Knowledge of the neural pathways for touch and pain allow neurologists to determine the location of damage to the nervous system. For example, if a patient has a complete loss of touch and pain on the right side of the body, there are only a few places where damage to the nervous system could cause this effect. It could not be caused by damage to a single nerve because damage to one nerve would produce localized sensory loss. Damage to the entire spinal cord cannot cause this effect because that would result in paralysis and loss of sensation on both sides of the body. Damage to just the right side of the spinal cord also is not an option because that would disrupt touch from the right leg and pain from the left leg. Damage to the cerebral cortex on the left side of the brain would cause a loss of touch and pain on the right, but it is unlikely that the entire somatosensory cortex would be damaged without damaging other parts of the brain. A patient with these symptoms probably has damage to the left side of the midbrain. The medial lemniscus and anterolateral pathways travel in the lateral midbrain and carry touch and pain from the right side of the body. Damage to these pathways will result in loss of both touch and pain on the right side. Although an understanding of neuroscience is valuable in and of itself, knowledge of the nervous system provides a powerful diagnostic tool to physicians treating neurological disorders.

LOCAL CONNECTIONS

The **medial longitudinal fasciculus** is a tight fiber bundle that connects nuclei controlling eye and head movements. It appears to merge with the trochlear nucleus as it makes connections with the various visual areas in the midbrain. These include the superior colliculus, pretectal area, oculomotor nucleus, and the trochlear nucleus. The medial longitudinal fasciculus also relays messages to and from the vestibular system, a series of structures involved in balance and head movements. Thus, the medial longitudinal fasciculus is critical in linking eye and head movements so objects can be followed.

The lateral lemniscus is difficult to see in cross sections of the midbrain because this fiber bundle terminates in the inferior colliculus, which is located at the border of the midbrain and pons. Auditory information ascending from the cochlear nucleus and superior olivary complex travels in the lateral lemniscus. The axons enter the inferior colliculus from the bottom along the lateral edge of the midbrain. This fiber tract is unique in that it carries information from both the right and left ears.

The transition from the midbrain to the thalamus is marked by a horizontally running fiber bundle called the **posterior commissure**. These axons appear as a white bar just above the aqueduct and in front of the superior colliculus. The posterior commissure runs horizontally because it connects neurons in the pretectal area on the right and left sides of the midbrain. Damage to these axons reduces the pupillary light reflex in the left eye when a light shines into the right eye (see "Pupillary Light Reflex" box in Chapter 5).

CRANIAL NERVES

Cranial nerves are unique in that these axons link brain nuclei with sensory systems and muscles on the head (Figure 8.2). Some cranial nerves carry sensory information into the brain

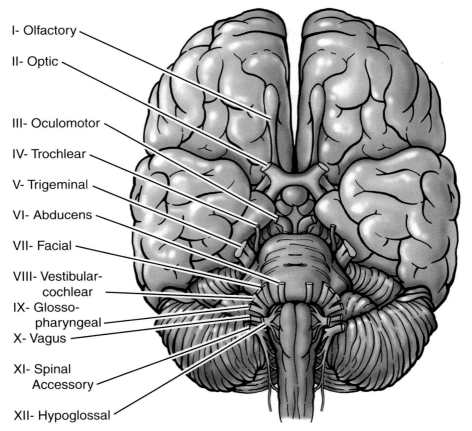

I- Olfactory

II- Optic

III- Oculomotor

IV- Trochlear

V- Trigeminal

VI- Abducens

VII- Facial

VIII- Vestibular-
     cochlear

IX- Glosso-
    pharyngeal

X- Vagus

XI- Spinal
    Accessory

XII- Hypoglossal

Figure 8.2 There are twelve pairs of cranial nerves. These nerves are involved in bringing sensory information to the brain and controlling the muscles of the head and neck. Two cranial nerves, the oculomotor and trochlear, originate from nuclei within the midbrain. These nerves control the muscles of the eye (see Chapter 5).

(e.g., cranial nerve II carries vision), others transmit commands to muscles (e.g., cranial nerve XI controls head and neck muscles), and some are both sensory and motor (e.g., cranial nerve VII carries taste and moves facial muscles).

Two cranial nerves exit at the level of the midbrain. The oculomotor (cranial nerve III) and trochlear (cranial nerve IV) nerves arise from the oculomotor and trochlear nuclei and project to the muscles that move the eyes. The oculomotor nerve descends through the middle of the midbrain between the red nuclei and exits the brain along the ventral surface. In contrast, the trochlear nerve is the only cranial nerve to exit the brain on the back side. These axons run between the inferior colliculi before leaving the brain. Damage to these nerves results in problems moving the eye.

SUMMARY

One of the most important functions of the midbrain is to serve as a conduit between the brain and the body. The largest axon bundles in the nervous system carry motor (cerebral peduncles) and tactile (medial lemniscus and anterolateral pathway) information through the midbrain. Smaller axon bundles carry information to and from the nuclei of the midbrain. If it were possible for the brain to go wireless and rid itself of all axons, the midbrain would shrink to one-fourth its current size. These nuclei are important, but without the axons, the neurons are worthless.

Glossary

Abducens a nucleus in the pons from which the abducens nerve (cranial nerve VI) originates. These neurons project to the lateral rectus muscle to turn the eye outward.

Amygdala a forebrain nucleus involved in emotions.

Analgesia a loss of sensitivity to pain.

Anterolateral pathway an axon bundle carrying pain sensations from the spinal cord to the thalamus.

Axon the part of a neuron extending from the cell body through which electrical signals are transmitted.

Basal ganglia a collection of forebrain nuclei (e.g., nucleus accumbens, striatum, globus pallidus) involved in motor control and other functions.

Basilar membrane the flexible inner ear membrane on which auditory hair cells sit.

Cerebellum large hindbrain structure involved in motor coordination.

Cerebral aqueduct a canal filled with cerebrospinal fluid that runs the length of the midbrain and connects the third and fourth ventricles.

Cerebral cortex the large and prominent neural covering of the forebrain.

Cerebral peduncle the large fiber bundle running along the bottom edge of the midbrain. Includes axons that make up the corticopontine, corticobulbar, and corticospinal tracts.

Ciliary ganglion a collection of neurons located between the brain and eye that control the size of the pupil and the shape of the lens.

Cochlea snail shell-shaped structure of the inner ear containing auditory hair cells.

Cochlear nucleus auditory nucleus in the medulla that receives input from the auditory nerve and projects to ascending auditory structures such as the superior olivary nucleus and inferior colliculus.

Coronal section a way to cut the brain into anterior and posterior parts.

Corticospinal tract a collection of axons involved in voluntary movement descending from the primary motor cortex to motoneurons in the spinal cord.

Cranial nerves the twelve pairs of nerves that enter and exit the brain directly.

Dendrite part of the neuron that receives and transmits messages to the cell body.

Dopamine a neurotransmitter produced by neurons located in the substantia nigra (movement) and ventral tegmental area (reward).

Dorsal column nuclei medullary nuclei that receive somatosensory input from the skin and project via the medial lemniscus to the thalamus.

Ganglion cells the output neurons of the retina that carry visual information to the thalamus and superior colliculus.

Glia a diverse collection of cells in the brain and spinal cord involved in maintaining the normal functioning of neurons.

Globus pallidus one of the nuclei of the basal ganglia involved in movement.

Hair cell a specialized auditory neuron in the inner ear that converts vibrations to neural activity.

Hippocampus a collection of forebrain neurons involved in memory formation.

Hypothalamus a part of the forebrain immediately anterior to the midbrain involved in many regulatory functions (e.g., body temperature, hunger, hormone levels).

Inferior colliculus a midbrain structure involved in auditory processing.

Interstitial nucleus of Cajal a midbrain structure that receives input about head movements so compensatory eye movements can be produced.

Lateral geniculate nucleus part of the thalamus that receives input from the retina and projects to the primary visual cortex.

Lateral lemniscus an axon bundle carrying auditory information from the cochlear nucleus and superior olivary complex to the inferior colliculus.

Medial forebrain bundle a bundle of axons running from the ventral tegmental area to the forebrain, stimulation of which is pleasurable (see Mesolimbic pathway).

Medial geniculate nucleus part of the thalamus that receives input from the inferior colliculus and projects to the primary auditory cortex.

Medial lemniscus an axon bundle carrying information about touch and joint position from the dorsal column nuclei in the medulla to the thalamus.

Medial longitudinal fasciculus a bundle of axons in the midbrain interconnecting nuclei involved in coordinating head and eye movements.

Medulla oblongata the part of the hindbrain located between the pons and spinal cord.

Mesencephalic reticular formation a loose collection of neurons in the midbrain involved in movement and other functions.

Mesolimbic pathway an axon tract involved in reward which projects from the ventral tegmental area to the forebrain.

Midsagittal section a way to cut the brain into identical right and left halves.

Motor system a diverse group of neural structures involved in movement.

Motoneuron specialized neurons projecting from the medulla and spinal cord which, when active, cause muscles to contract.

Neurons the cells of the nervous system involved in transmitting messages from one place to another. A typical neuron has dendrites, a cell body, and an axon.

Neurotransmitter the chemical messenger released by the axon of a neuron.

Nucleus accumbens the basal ganglia nucleus involved in reward.

Nucleus the general name for a collection of neurons in the brain or spinal cord (e.g., substantia nigra, red nucleus).

Occipital cortex the part of the cerebral cortex located at the back of the brain. This region process visual images for conscious awareness.

Oculomotor nucleus a midbrain structure that controls four eye muscles by way of the oculomotor nerve (Cranial nerve III).

Opioid the name of a group of naturally occurring neurotransmitters (enkephalin, endorphin, dynorphin) involved in pain inhibition.

Optic tectum neurons along the top of the midbrain involved in processing visual motion. Called the superior colliculus in humans.

Periaqueductal gray (PAG) a collection of neurons involved in defense surrounding the cerebral aqueduct in the midbrain.

Pons part of the hindbrain located between the midbrain and medulla oblongata. The cerebellum is attached to the pons via the cerebellar peduncles.

Posterior commissure a small bundle of axons at the anterior edge of the midbrain connecting structures on the right and left sides of the midbrain.

Prefrontal cortex part of the cerebral cortex located at the front of the brain. Involved in decision making.

Pretectal area midbrain neurons involved in visual reflexes located immediately anterior to the superior colliculus.

Primary motor cortex the group of neurons involved in voluntary movement located at the top of the cerebral cortex. These neurons are the source of the corticospinal tract.

Purkinje cells the only neurons that send signals away from the cerebellum. Discovered by Johannes Evangelista Purkinje.

Receptor a protein located on the surface of a neuron to which neurotransmitter binds.

Red nucleus a midbrain structure involved in learned movements.

Reticular formation a diffuse collection of neurons located in the bottom half of the midbrain, pons, and medulla.

Reticulospinal tract a collection of axons involved in movement descending from the reticular formation to the spinal cord.

Rostral ventromedial medulla (RVM) a collection of neurons in the medulla involved in pain modulation that receive input from the periaqueductal gray.

Rubrospinal tract a collection of axons involved in movement descending from the red nucleus to the spinal cord.

Sensorimotor cortex part of the cerebral cortex located at the top of the brain involved in integrating sensory input and motor output.

Somatosensation those sensations arising from the skin (i.e., touch, temperature, pain).

Striatum the basal ganglia nucleus that receives input from the substantia nigra in order to initiate movement.

Substantia nigra a dark-colored nucleus in the midbrain that contains dopamine and is involved in initiating movement.

Superior cerebellar peduncle a bundle of axons carrying motor signals from the cerebellum through the midbrain to the thalamus.

Superior colliculus a collection of neurons in the midbrain involved in coordinating eye and head movements.

Superior olivary complex a collection of neurons in the medulla that receives input from both ears and is involved in localizing sounds.

Tectorial membrane the rigid membrane in the cochlea that cause the stereocilia on hair cells to bend in order to code sound.

Thalamus part of the forebrain immediately above the hypothalamus and anterior to the midbrain.

Tonotopic map the organization of neurons in auditory structures (e.g., inferior colliculus) whereby adjacent neurons code similar sound frequencies.

Torus semicircularis a collection of midbrain neurons involved in auditory processing and/or electroreception. These neurons are called the inferior colliculus in humans.

Tract the general name for a collection of axons traveling through the brain and/or spinal cord together (e.g., corticospinal tract).

Trochlear nucleus a midbrain structure that gives rise to the trochlear nerve (Cranial nerve IV) which controls the superior oblique muscle of the eye.

Ventral tegmental area (VTA) a midbrain nucleus made up of dopamine-containing neurons involved in reward.

Vestibular nuclei a collection of hindbrain nuclei that code head position and movement.

Vestibulospinal tract a collection of axons involved in movement descending from the vestibular nuclei to the spinal cord.

Bibliography

Amano, K., et al. "Single Neuron Analysis of the Human Midbrain Tegumentum." *Applied Neurophysiology* 41 (1982): 66–67.

Blumenfeld, H. *Neuroanatomy Through Clinical Cases.* Sunderland, MA: Sinauer Associates, 2002.

Butler, A. B., and W. Hodos. *Comparative Vertebrate Neuroanatomy: Evolution and Adaptation.* New York: Wiley-Liss, Inc., 1996.

Hendelman, W. J. *Atlas of Functional Neuroanatomy.* Boca Raton, FL: CRC Press, 2000.

Johnstone, A. "So, What's Really Going on in Those Young Heads? They May Look Like Adults, but Don't be Fooled. New Studies Show the Brain is Such a Cauldron of Activity that our Teenagers are Far from Mature." *The Herald* (UK) Jan 10, 2004: 4.

Kandel, E. R., J. H., Schwartz, and T. M. Jessell (Editors). *Principles of Neural Science, 4th ed.* New York: McGraw-Hill, 2000.

Langston J. W., P. Ballard, J. W. Tetrud, and I. Irwin. "Chronic Parkinsonism in Humans due to a Product of Meperidine-analog Synthesis." *Science* 219 (1983): 979–980.

Langston, J. W., and J. Palfreman. *The Case of the Frozen Addicts.* New York: Pantheon Books, 1995.

Marshall, L. H., and H. W. Magoun. *Discoveries in the Human Brain: Neuroscience Prehistory, Brain Structure, and Function.* Totowa, NJ: Humana Press, 1998.

Nashold, B. S., Jr., et al. "Sensations Evoked by Stimulation of the Midbrain of Man." *Journal of Neurosugery* 30 (1969): 14–24.

Nestler, E. J., and R. C. Malenka. "The addicted brain." *Scientific American* (March 2004): 78–85.

Paxinos, G., and J. K. Mai (Editors). *The Human Nervous System, 2nd ed.* San Diego: Academic Press, 2003.

Squire, L. R., et al. *Fundamental Neuroscience, 2nd ed.* San Diego: Academic Press, 2003.

Further Reading

Carter, R. *Mapping the Mind.* Berkeley, CA: University of California Press, 1998.

Greenfield, S. A. *The Human Brain: A Guided Tour.* Science Masters series, New York: Basic Books, 1997.

LeDoux, Jh. *The Emotional Brain: The Mysterious Underpinnings of Emotional Life.* New York: Touchstone Books, 1998.

Nolte, J., and J. B. Angevine. *The Human Brain*, Mosby, 1995.

Ramachandran, V. S., and S. Blakeslee. *Phantoms in the Brain: Probing the Mysteries of the Human Mind.* New York: William Morrow & Company, 1998.

Sanes, D. H., T. A. Reh, and W. A. Harris, eds. *Development of the Nervous System.* New York: Academic Press, 2000.

Web Sites

Divisions of the Nervous System
http://faculty.washington.edu/chudler/nsdivide.html

Neuroscience Terminology
http://serendip.brynmawr.edu/bb/kinser/Glossary.html

Mammalian Brain Collections
http://brainmuseum.org/

Brain Evolution
http://brainmuseum.org/Evolution/

Neuroscience History Articles
http://www.ibro.org/Pub_Main_Display.asp?Main_ID511

Milestones in Neuroscience
http://faculty.washington.edu/chudler/hist.html

UCLA Archive on Pain and Suffering
http://www.library.ucla.edu/libraries/biomed/his/painexhibit/ index.html

National Institute on Deafness and other Communication Disorders
http://www.nidcd.nih.gov/

National Institute on Neurological Disorders and Stroke
http://www.ninds.nih.gov/

National Eye Institute
http://www.nei.nih.gov/

National Institute on Drug Abuse
http://www.nida.nih.gov/

The Science Underlying Drug Abuse
http://www.teens.drugabuse.gov/

Index

Abducens nuclei
function, 54, 58, 60, 99
ADHD. *See* Attention deficit
hyperactivity disorder
Amygdala, 2
function, 68, 70, 75–76, 81,
83–84, 99
Analgesia, 99
and defense response, 66–73, 77
opioids, 69, 71–75, 77, 102
Anterolateral pathway, 94–95, 98–99
Aristotle, 10
Attention deficit hyperactivity
disorder (ADHD), 27
Auditory cortex
function, 46–48, 101
neurons in, 39, 41–42
Auditory nerve, 38, 41–42, 47, 99
Auditory system, 75, 96
localization, 43, 103
loss of, 37, 44
sound processing, 4, 13–14,
18–19, 21, 28, 35–49, 54, 82,
100, 103
Axon
function, 8–12, 33, 79, 81–82,
90–91, 93–94, 96, 98–104
myelin sheath, 8, 91

Basal ganglia, 1
function, 28–29, 55, 79, 99–100,
102–3
structures in, 26–28
Basilar membrane
function, 37–39, 41, 99
Bat sonar, 39–40
Blind sight, 51–52
Brain, 100
anatomy, 1–8, 10, 12, 16, 22,
24–25, 27, 29–32, 41, 46,
48–49, 52, 56, 68, 78–79,
81–82, 90–92, 102–4

damage, 10, 25, 52
function, 16, 22, 25, 28, 43,
45–46, 51–52, 96–99
research, 10, 12, 69, 88
size, 14–15, 17, 22
Brain stem, 5
functions, 30
Broca, Paul, 10

Cell body, 2, 65
function, 8–9, 11, 99, 100–1
Cerebellum
function, 32, 55, 94–95,
99, 103
location, 2–3, 5, 44–45, 102
Cerebral aqueduct
function, 65, 96, 99, 102
location, 5–6, 8, 19
Cerebral cortex, 1
damage, 95
functions, 15–16, 28, 31, 41, 43,
47, 63, 68, 75, 91, 102–3
location, 2–6, 44–45, 99
occipital lobe, 51
size, 14, 17
temporal lobes of, 2, 83
Cerebral peduncle
damage to, 94
function, 95, 98
location, 91, 93, 99, 102
superior, 7
Ciliary ganglion, 57, 61–62, 99
Cochlea
nucleus, 41–42, 44, 47, 96,
99, 101
stereocilia in, 37–38, 41, 103
Comparative neuroanatomy,
13–22
Coronal section, 5–6, 19, 26, 29,
93, 100
Corticospinal tract, 10
and movement, 30, 32–33,
93–94, 99–100, 102–3

Cranial nerves, 100
    function, 53, 57–59, 96–98,
        102, 104
Crux cerebri, 8

Defense behaviors, 1, 49, 64
    analgesia, 66–75, 77, 99, 102
    escape and survival, 48,
        67–68, 70
    flight or fight response, 66–68,
        70, 77
    immobility, 48, 66, 70, 77
    physiological changes, 65–68,
        76, 83
Dendrite
    function, 8–9, 11, 100–1
Deoxyribonucleic acid (DNA), 8–9
Descartes René, 92
Diencephalon. See Forebrain
Diplopia, 61
DNA. See Deoxyribonucleic acid
Dopamine
    function, 25–27, 103
    production, 6, 11, 25, 27, 79–80,
        85–88, 100, 104
    related disorders, 25, 27
Dorsal column nuclei, 44, 94, 100–1
Drug abuse
    and opiates, 74, 85–88
    and reward pathway, 85–89

Edinger-Westphal nucleus
    function, 53, 56–57, 61–62
Electroreception, 13, 19, 21, 104

Forebrain (Diencephalon and
        Telencephalon)
    function, 14, 18, 33
    location, 3, 14
    size, 16
    structures, 1, 26–27, 29, 70,
        75–76, 78–79, 82–83, 99–101,
        103

Galen, 10
Galvani, Luigi, 10
Ganglion cells
    in the retina, 54, 57, 100
Glia, 8–9, 100
Globus pallidus
    function, 25, 28–29, 44, 46,
        99–100

Hindbrain (Metencephalon), 1
    location, 2, 4, 14, 102
    structures, 3, 99, 101, 104
Hippocampus, 2, 81, 83–84, 100
Hypoglossal nerve, 58
Hypothalamus
    functions, 1, 3–4, 68, 75–76,
        100, 103

Inferior colliculus
    anatomy of, 44–46
    damage to, 44
    function, 14, 18, 21, 35, 40–42,
        44, 46–49, 75–76, 96,
        98–101, 103
    location, 6–7, 20–21, 41,
        44–45, 54
    pathway from the ear, 41–44
    size, 18
    and sound, 35–49
Interstitial nucleus of Cajal
    function, 51, 54, 61–63, 100

Lateral geniculate nucleus
    function, 55–57, 101
    location, 51
Lateral lemniscus, 93, 96
    nuclei, 41–42, 101
Lateral PAG
    defense response, 68, 77
    location, 65

Medial forebrain bundle
    stimulation of, 80–82, 101

Medial geniculate nucleus
    function, 41–42, 48, 101
Medial lemniscus, 93–95, 98, 100–1
Medial longitudinal fasciculus
    function, 53, 59, 96, 101
Medulla oblongata, 33
    functions, 44, 54–55, 75, 91,
        101–2
    location, 2–3, 5–6
    structures in, 41–42, 94, 99–101,
        103
Mesencephalic reticular formation,
    8, 101
Mesencephalon. See Midbrain
Mesolimbic pathway
    and reward, 79–81, 85, 87–88,
        101
Metencephalon. See Hindbrain
Midbrain (Mesencephalon)
    functions, 1, 6, 8, 12, 14, 16,
        33–34, 51–53, 98
    location, 2–4, 14, 18–19
    size, 14–15, 17–19
    structures, 2–12, 14, 16–22, 24,
        26–27, 31–32, 35, 41, 44–45,
        49–55, 57–63, 65–67, 75–76,
        78–80, 91, 93–104
Midsagittal section, 3, 5, 17, 76,
    101
Milner, Peter, 82
Motoneuron, 8
    and muscle contraction, 28, 30,
        32–33, 94, 100–1
Motor systems, 1, 32, 57, 101, 103
Movement
    control of, 23–34, 44, 46, 93–97,
        99–100, 103–4
    disorders, 23–28, 34
    eye and head, 50–61, 63, 80,
        96–98, 100–3
    involuntary, 55, 59
    learned automatic, 24, 33, 103
    reflexes, 24, 32

voluntary circuit, 24, 28–33, 55,
    79, 94, 100, 102
Multiple sclerosis, 91

Neuron
    communication, 11–12
    functions, 8–9, 11–12, 18,
        24–28, 32–33, 37–41, 43–44,
        46–48, 52, 54, 56, 68, 72–74,
        76–77, 79, 81–85, 88, 90–91,
        94, 96, 98–104
    parts, 8–12, 28, 102
    in retina, 54, 56, 61–62
    types, 8, 24–26, 28, 46, 86
Nervous system
    autonomic, 75
    disorders, 26, 95
    peripheral, 74
    structures, 1, 9–10, 24, 30, 32, 41,
        72, 74, 76, 87, 90, 95, 98, 101
Neuroscience, 10, 49
    research, 69, 84, 95
Neurotransmitter
    types, 6, 11–12, 25–27, 37, 38, 41,
        71, 75, 79–80, 85, 100, 102
Nucleus accumbens, 2
    and the reward pathway, 78–88,
        99, 102

Occipital cortex
    function, 18, 102
Oculomotor nuclei, 93
    damage to, 52, 59
    function, 4, 6, 34, 51, 53–55,
        58–61, 63, 90, 96–98, 102
Olds, James, 82
Opiates, 102
    addictive properties, 72, 85–88
    side effects, 72, 74
    uses, 71–72, 77
Opioid receptors
    analgesia, 69, 71–75, 101–2
Optic nerve, 57, 62

Optic tectum, 18–21, 56, 102
Optokinetic reflex, 56

PAG. *See* Periaqueductal gray
Parkinson's disease
    causes, 24, 26, 27, 32
    characteristics of, 23–25
    treatment, 23
Periaqueductal gray (PAG)
    function, 49, 59, 65–77, 81,
        102–3
    location, 6–8, 54, 65
    structures, 65–66
Piloerection, 66
Pons, 33
    location, 2–6, 45, 102
    structures in, 60, 91, 94, 96,
        99, 101
Posterior commissure, 93, 96, 102
Prefrontal cortex
    functions, 76, 79, 83–84, 102
Premotor cortex, 28
Pretectal area
    location, 56, 62
    function, 48, 54–57, 62, 96, 102
Primary motor cortex, 100, 102
    damage to, 31
    function, 28, 30, 32–33, 94–95
Primary visual cortex, 52,
    55–57, 100
Pupillary light reflex, 56–57, 61, 96
Purkinje cells, 8, 102

Receptors
    neurotransmitter, 11, 102
Red nucleus, 9, 18
    function, 31–34, 103
    location, 6–8, 19, 20, 26, 31 98,
        103
Reticulospinal tract
    and movement, 30–32, 103
Reward behaviors, 1
    and addiction, 85–89

inherent, 82
learned, 82
pathway, 78–87, 100, 102, 104
Rostral ventromedial medulla
    (RVM)
    function, 71–76, 103
Rubrospinal tract
    and movement, 30–33, 103
RVM. *See* Rostral ventromedial
    medulla

Saccadic eye movements, 56, 59
Schizophrenia, 27
Schwann, Theodor, 10
Sensory processes, 1
    feedback, 30–32, 94, 96, 103
    hearing, 4, 13–14, 18–19, 21, 28,
        35–49, 54, 75, 100–1, 103
    sight, 4, 13–14, 16, 18–19, 21,
        28, 48–63, 75, 82, 102
    smell, 13–14, 21, 28, 57
    touch and taste, 21, 28, 46, 49,
        54, 57, 82
Sensorimotor cortex, 31, 103
Serotonin, 11
Somatosensation, 54, 95, 100, 103
Spinal accessory nerve, 58
Spinal cord, 1–2, 6, 103
    functions, 28, 30, 32–33, 55, 68,
        72–76, 91, 94–95, 99–101, 104
Striatum, 79–80, 99, 103
Substantia nigra
    function, 6, 24–26, 29, 32, 44,
        46, 55, 72, 80–81, 103
    location, 6–8, 26–28, 31, 79,
        91, 100
    parts, 25
Superior cerebellar peduncle
    location, 7, 94–95, 103
Superior colliculus
    damage to, 52
    function, 48–63, 75–76, 80, 96,
        100, 102–3

location, 6–7, 20–21, 44–45, 54
    size, 18
Superior oblique muscle, 59
Superior olivary complex
    function, 41–43, 46–47, 96, 99,
        101, 103
Striatum, 2, 28–29

Tectorial membrane
    in the cochlea, 37, 103
Telencephalon. *See* Forebrain
Thalamus
    function, 29
    location, 1–2, 5, 28, 45, 103
    structures of, 41–42, 51, 55, 57,
        94–96, 99–101, 103
Tonotopic map, 39, 44, 49, 103
Torus semicircularis, 18–21, 104
Tourette's syndrome, 27
Tract
    examples, 10, 30–33, 90, 93–94,
        99, 102, 104

Trochlear nuclei, 61, 103
    damage to, 59
    function, 4, 6, 34, 51, 53–55,
        58–60, 63, 96–98, 104

Ventral tegmental area (VTA)
    function, 6, 78–88, 100–1, 104
    location, 6, 8, 27, 78–80, 91
Ventrolateral PAG
    defense response, 72, 77
    location, 65
Vestibular nuclei, 61, 104
Vestibulospinal tract, 104
    and movement, 30, 32
Vision
    pathways, 54–56, 75
    peripheral, 54, 66
    sight, 4, 13–14, 16, 18–19, 21,
        28, 48–63, 102
    structures, 52–58
    systems, 51–53, 57, 63
VTA. *See* Ventral tegmental area

About the Author

Michael Morgan is professor of psychology at Washington State University, Vancouver. His interest in neuroscience was triggered by a physiological psychology course he took during his sophomore year at UCLA. Two years later (1984), he graduated with a B.A. degree in psychology and began graduate training the following semester at UCLA under the supervision of Dr. John Liebeskind. Dr. Morgan graduated with a Ph.D. in physiological psychology from UCLA in 1989, winning both the Joseph A. Gengerelli Distinguished Dissertation Award and the Shephard Ivory Franz Outstanding Teaching Award. Dr. Morgan continued his training at UCSF as a post-doctoral fellow under the supervision of Dr. Howard Fields.

In 1993, Dr. Morgan accepted a position as assistant professor of psychology at Washington State University, Vancouver. He has continued to find success with both teaching and research, earning the Students' Award for Teaching Excellence in 1997, the James F. Adams Excellence in Graduate Education Award in 2003, and the Chancellor's Award for Research Excellence in 2004. He was promoted to full professor in 2005. Dr. Morgan's research is funded by the National Institute on Drug Abuse and focuses on the contribution of the periaqueductal gray to tolerance to the analgesic effects of morphine. When not at work, Dr. Morgan keeps his mind and body active by reading, running, and hiking.

■ Picture Credits